Updates in Surgery

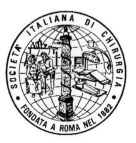

Paolo Pederzoli • Claudio Bassi
Editors

Uncommon Pancreatic Neoplasms

In collaboration with
Massimo Falconi, Roberto Salvia and Giovanni Butturini

Foreword by
Gianluigi Melotti

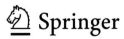

Editors
Paolo Pederzoli
Department of Surgery and Oncology
General Surgery Unit, Pancreas Center
"G.B. Rossi" University Hospital
Verona, Italy

Claudio Bassi
Department of Surgery and Oncology
General Surgery Unit, Pancreas Center
"G.B. Rossi" University Hospital
Verona, Italy

In collaboration with:
Massimo Falconi, Roberto Salvia and Giovanni Butturini

The publication and the distribution of this volume have been supported by the Italian Society of Surgery

ISSN 2280-9848
ISBN 978-88-470-2672-8   e-ISBN 978-88-470-2673-5

DOI 10.1007/978-88-470-2673-5

Springer Milan Dordrecht Heidelberg London New York

Library of Congress Control Number: 2012944071

© Springer-Verlag Italia 2013

This work is subject to copyright. All rights are reserved by the Publisher, whether the whole or part of the material is concerned, specifically the rights of translation, reprinting, reuse of illustrations, recitation, broadcasting, reproduction on microfilms or in any other physical way, and transmission or information storage and retrieval, electronic adaptation, computer software, or by similar or dissimilar methodology now known or hereafter developed. Exempted from this legal reservation are brief excerpts in connection with reviews or scholarly analysis or material supplied specifically for the purpose of being entered and executed on a computer system, for exclusive use by the purchaser of the work. Duplication of this publication or parts thereof is permitted only under the provisions of the Copyright Law of the Publisher's location, in its current version, and permission for use must always be obtained from Springer. Permissions for use may be obtained through RightsLink at the Copyright Clearance Center. Violations are liable to prosecution under the respective Copyright Law.

The use of general descriptive names, registered names, trademarks, service marks, etc. in this publication does not imply , even in the absence of a specific statement, that such names are exempt from the relevant protective laws and regulations and therefore free for general use.

While the advice and information in this book are believed to be true and accurate at the date of publication, neither the authors nor the editors nor the publisher can accept any legal responsibility for any errors or omissions that may be made. The publisher makes no warranty, express or implied, with respect to the material contained herein.

9 8 7 6 5 4 3 2 1   2013   2014   2015   2016

Cover design: Ikona S.r.l., Milan, Italy
Typesetting: Graphostudio, Milan, Italy
Printing and binding: Arti Grafiche Nidasio S.r.l., Assago, Italy

Printed in Italy

Springer-Verlag Italia S.r.l. – Via Decembrio 28 – I-20137 Milan
Springer is a part of Springer Science+Business Media (www.springer.com)

Foreword

It gives me great pleasure to introduce this comprehensive and exceptionally informative book on uncommon pancreatic neoplasms, including cystic, endocrine, and unusual solid tumors.

Although individually they are deemed "uncommon", viewed together these neoplasms are of very high clinical interest and importance. Furthermore, advances in imaging have made it possible to detect small lesions in the pancreas in asymptomatic patients, and the neoplasms discussed in this volume can frequently be treated by surgery alone or by a multimodal approach with curative intent.

In bringing together Italian experts in pathology, imaging, surgery, and medical oncology to write this book, the editors, Professors Paolo Pederzoli and Claudio Bassi, have aimed to provide an integrated coverage that will acquaint clinicians and surgeons more closely with the described pathologies, reflecting their complexity and highlighting the state of the art in diagnosis and treatment, both surgical and medical. Without doubt they have succeeded in this goal! All aspects, from clinical presentation, genetics, and pathology through to diagnostic imaging, treatment, and follow-up, are considered with the degree of care expected by the discerning reader.

It is my belief that the wide range of specialists involved in the care of patients with the described neoplasms will benefit enormously from this book, which provides all the tools needed for modern pathological classification and clinical management of these patients. Optimal surgical treatment is certainly based upon such a thorough multidisciplinary approach.

My congratulations to Paolo and Claudio for this fine achievement!

Rome, September 2012

Gianluigi Melotti
President, Italian Society of Surgery

Preface

It is with a true sense of delight that I offer readers this book on rare pancreatic neoplasms. When the director of the Italian Society of Surgery (SIC) and my good friend Dr. Melotti invited me to choose a topic related to pancreatology as the subject of a book, I decided to focus on rare pancreatic neoplasms rather than on pancreatic ductal adenocarcinoma.

The term "rare," as referred to pancreatic neoplasms, has recently become a matter of discussion, since the widespread use of more sophisticated imaging technologies has resulted in the detection of an increasing number of asymptomatic lesions in the pancreas. More frequently, these lesions are cystic in nature; only a few of them are neoplasms harboring malignant potential. Given that most of these conditions are scarcely known from a biological standpoint, their clinical management is challenging and highly debated.

This book is divided into three parts, covering: cystic pancreatic neoplasms, neuroendocrine pancreatic neoplasms, and uncommon pancreatic solid neoplasms. Each section has been coordinated by an experienced pancreatic surgeon from our Surgical Department who is recognized for his expertise in the respective area. This experience has been broadened through collaborations with specialists from numerous other fields, including gastroenterologists, pathologists, oncologists, radiologists, and molecular biologists. Not surprisingly, the integration of these perspectives has been very successful, since multidisciplinarity is one of the main strengths of the Verona pancreatic group.

The primary goal of this book is to offer readers a thorough, useful, readable, and understandable manual that presents an overview of rare pancreatic neoplasms and emphasizes the need for their multidisciplinary management. It is designed for rapid consultation whether by students, trainees, or experts in the field.

I would like to thank Prof. Claudio Bassi in particular for joining me with great enthusiasm in the supervision of this book's preparation. I also thank the coordinators of each section, Prof. Massimo Falconi, Prof. Roberto Salvia, and Dr. Giovanni Butturini, for their excellent work.

Finally, my appreciation is directed at all the coauthors involved in this project, for their helpfulness and remarkable dedication to the creation of an accessible, unique and up-to-date manual.

I believe this collective effort will long serve as a valuable resource for readers interested in broadening their knowledge of some of the most fascinating and challenging topics in modern pancreatology.

Verona, September 2012   Paolo Pederzoli

Preface

It was during the early 1970s that Dr. Pederzoli, recently graduated from the prestigious University of Padua, decided to follow Professor Adamo Dagradi to the newly founded University of Verona. According to local legend, Paolo Pederzoli made this move since he had heard that in the city of Romeo and Juliet he would be able to focus on the pancreas. The same legend reports that the young pupil had to first ask his mentor: "Ok, so where is the pancreas?".

Many years have passed since that day, and time has flowed "like the water of the Adige River, where it makes a "U" turn in the city of Verona, as if it did not want to leave its beauty" (Berto Barbarani, Verona's most famous poet).

That same Paolo Pederzoli who has never left his adopted city, has converted his devotion to the pancreas into a stunning professional career, recognized at the highest levels not only in Italy but also abroad. The "secret" of this success is contained in the following pages, which reveal a thorough and exhaustive knowledge of pancreatic diseases, including discussions of uncommon lesions rarely seen outside high-volume centers, and the logic underlying the adoption of a multidisciplinary approach to their diagnosis and management.

This book presents the most recent findings on cystic, neuroendocrine, and other uncommon pancreatic neoplasms, with particular emphasis on their surgical pathology. A decision-making algorithm for each entity is provided in detail, while the above-mentioned multidisciplinary approach encompasses issues related to a variety of specialties, such as gastroenterology, oncology, endocrinology, and molecular biology. Clearly, this manual offers specialists in different areas of pancreatology a unique guide to uncommon pancreatic diseases.

But are these diseases really "uncommon"? Certainly, a high-volume tertiary care center, such as the one directed for decades by Professor Pederzoli, cannot be considered representative of the "outside" reality. On the other hand, it is surprising how often a radiologist from a low-volume hospital must deal with small and asymptomatic pancreatic cysts. Our knowledge of these cysts has advanced to the stage that they can be regarded as extraordinary in vivo models whose developing pattern can be clinically monitored.

It is not only the morphologic features distinguished using sophisticated imaging techniques that have improved our understanding of pancreatic diseases. Tremendous advances also have been made in elucidating both the carcinogenic pathways that result in cystic neoplasms such as intraductal papillary mucinous neoplasms and the complex biology of neuroendocrine tumors.

Collectively, a deeper understanding of these uncommon diseases, some of which are precursor lesions of ductal adenocarcinoma, will equip us with crucial models that can be applied to unravel the biology of their more frequently occurring malignant counterparts.

Professor Pederzoli concludes his academic career by having involved all of his closest collaborators and colleagues in the creation of this valuable work: Thank you Paolo for your enthusiasm and for your passionate dedication to the challenging task of assembling this book. Your leadership, intense determination, and deep commitment to this wonderful profession that you have chosen will continue to inspire us in our own careers.

Verona, September 2012   Claudio Bassi

Contents

Part I
Cystic Pancreatic Neoplasms 1
Roberto Salvia

1 Classification 3
Giuseppe Zamboni

2 Serous Cystic Neoplasms 5
Giuseppe Malleo, Giuseppe Zamboni, Marina Paini,
Giovanni Marchegiani and Riccardo Manfredi

3 Mucinous Cystic Neoplasms 15
Giovanni Marchegiani, Riccardo Manfredi, Giuseppe Malleo,
Isabella Frigerio and Giuseppe Zamboni

4 Solid-pseudopapillary, Acinar, and Other Cystic Neoplasms 23
Marina Paini, Giuseppe Zamboni, Riccardo Manfredi,
Salvatore Paiella and Giuseppe Malleo

5 Intraductal Papillary Mucinous Neoplasms 33
Isabella Frigerio, Giuseppe Zamboni, Riccardo Manfredi, Antonio Pea,
Silvia Pennacchio, Eugene Lim and Roberto Salvia

6 The Role of the Oncologist in the Diagnosis and Management
of Malignant Cystic Neoplasms 53
Alessandra Auriemma, Davide Melisi and Giampaolo Tortora

Part II
Neuroendocrine Pancreatic Neoplasms 59
Massimo Falconi

7 Epidemiology and Clinical Presentation 61
Maria Vittoria Davì, Marco Toaiari and Giuseppe Francia

8 Pathology and Genetics 71
Aldo Scarpa and Vincenzo Corbo

9 Imaging 79
Roberto Pozzi Mucelli, Giovanni Foti and Luigi Romano

10 Surgical Therapy 109
Rossella Bettini, Stefano Partelli, Stefano Crippa, Letizia Boninsegna
and Massimo Falconi

**11 Functional Imaging and Peptide Receptor
Radionuclide Therapy** 117
Maria Chiara Ambrosetti, Duccio Volterrani, Federica Guidoccio,
Lisa Bodei, Federica Orsini, Giuliano Mariani and Marco Ferdeghini

12 Targeted and Other Non-receptor-mediated Therapies 135
Sara Cingarlini, Chiara Trentin, Elisabetta Grego and Giampaolo Tortora

Part III
Uncommon Pancreatic Solid Neoplasms 147
Giovanni Butturini

13 Rare Variants of Ductal Adenocarcinoma of the Pancreas 149
Paolo Regi, Marco Dal Molin, Federica Pedica, Paola Capelli,
Mirko D'Onofrio and Giovanni Butturini

14 Rare Primary Tumors of the Pancreas 159
Marco Dal Molin, Paola Capelli, Mirko D'Onofrio, Ivana Cataldo,
Giovanni Marchegiani and Giovanni Butturini

15 Rare Secondary Tumors of the Pancreas 175
Giovanni Butturini, Marco Inama, Marco Dal Molin, Mirko D'Onofrio,
Davide Melisi, Giampaolo Tortora, Federica Pedica and Paola Capelli

16 Primary Non-epithelial Tumors of the Pancreas 189
Marco Dal Molin and Paola Capelli

17 Tumor-like Lesions of the Pancreas 193

Luca Frulloni, Antonio Amodio, Italo Vantini, Marco Dal Molin, Marco Inama, Mirko D'Onofrio, Lisa Marcolini, Claudio Luchini, Giovanni Butturini and Paola Capelli

Index 207

Contributors

Maria Chiara Ambrosetti Department of Pathology and Diagnostics, "G.B. Rossi" University Hospital, Verona, Italy

Antonio Amodio Department of Medicine, Pancreas Center, "G.B. Rossi" University Hospital, Verona, Italy

Alessandra Auriemma Department of Medical Oncology, "G.B. Rossi" University Hospital, Verona, Italy

Claudio Bassi Department of Surgery and Oncology, General Surgery Unit, Pancreas Center, "G.B. Rossi" University Hospital, Verona, Italy

Rossella Bettini Department of Surgery and Oncology, "G.B. Rossi" University Hospital, Verona, Italy and General Surgery Unit, "Sacro Cuore – Don Calabria" Hospital, Negrar (VR), Italy

Lisa Bodei Division of Nuclear Medicine, European Institute of Oncology, Milan, Italy

Letizia Boninsegna Department of Surgery and Oncology, "G.B. Rossi" University Hospital, Verona, Italy and General Surgery Unit, "Sacro Cuore – Don Calabria" Hospital, Negrar (VR), Italy

Giovanni Butturini Department of Surgery and Oncology, General Surgery Unit, Pancreas Center, "G.B. Rossi" University Hospital, Verona, Italy

Paola Capelli Department of Pathology and Diagnostics, Pathology Unit, "G.B. Rossi" University Hospital, Verona, Italy

Ivana Cataldo Department of Pathology and Diagnostics, Pathology Unit, "G.B. Rossi" University Hospital, Verona, Italy

Sara Cingarlini Department of Medical Oncology, "G.B. Rossi" University Hospital, Verona, Italy

Vincenzo Corbo Department of Pathology and Diagnostics, Pathology Unit, "G.B. Rossi" University Hospital and ARC-NET Research Centre, University of Verona, Verona, Italy

Stefano Crippa Department of Surgery and Oncology, "G.B. Rossi" University Hospital, Verona, Italy and General Surgery Unit, "Sacro Cuore – Don Calabria" Hospital, Negrar (VR), Italy

Marco Dal Molin Department of Surgery and Oncology, General Surgery Unit, Pancreas Center, "G.B. Rossi" University Hospital, Verona, Italy

Maria Vittoria Davì Department of Internal Medicine, "G.B. Rossi" University Hospital, Verona, Italy

Mirko D'Onofrio Department of Pathology and Diagnostics, Radiology Unit, "G.B. Rossi" University Hospital, Verona, Italy

Massimo Falconi Department of Surgery and Oncology, "G.B. Rossi" University Hospital, Verona, Italy and General Surgery Unit, "Sacro Cuore – Don Calabria" Hospital, Negrar (VR), Italy

Marco Federghini Department of Pathology and Diagnostics, Radiology Unit, "G.B. Rossi" University Hospital, Verona, Italy

Giovanni Foti Radiology Unit, "Sacro Cuore - Don Calabria" Hospital, Negrar (VR), Italy

Giuseppe Francia Department of Internal Medicine, "G.B. Rossi" University Hospital, Verona, Italy

Isabella Frigerio Surgery Unit, Casa di cura "Dr. P. Pederzoli", Peschiera del Garda (VR), Italy

Luca Frulloni Department of Medicine, Pancreas Center, "G.B. Rossi" University Hospital, Verona, Italy

Elisabetta Greco Department of Medical Oncology, "G.B. Rossi" University Hospital, Verona, Italy

Federica Guidoccio Regional Center of Nuclear Medicine, University of Pisa Medical School, Pisa, Italy

Marco Inama Department of Surgery and Oncology, General Surgery Unit, Pancreas Center, "G.B. Rossi" University Hospital, Verona, Italy

Eugene Lim National University of Singapore

Claudio Luchini Department of Pathology and Diagnostics, Pathology Unit, "G.B. Rossi" University Hospital, Verona, Italy

Giuseppe Malleo Department of Surgery and Oncology, General Surgery Unit, Pancreas Center, "G.B. Rossi" University Hospital, Verona, Italy

Riccardo Manfredi Department of Pathology and Diagnostics, Radiology Unit, "G.B. Rossi" University Hospital, Verona, Italy

Giovanni Marchegiani Department of Surgery and Oncology, General Surgery Unit, Pancreas Center, "G.B. Rossi" University Hospital, Verona, Italy

Lisa Marcolini Department of Pathology and Diagnostics, Pathology Unit, "G.B. Rossi" University Hospital, Verona, Italy

Giuliano Mariani Regional Center of Nuclear Medicine, University of Pisa Medical School, Pisa, Italy

Davide Melisi Department of Medical Oncology, "G.B. Rossi" University Hospital, Verona, Italy

Federica Orsini Regional Center of Nuclear Medicine, University of Pisa Medical School, Pisa, Italy

Salvatore Paiella Department of Surgery and Oncology, General Surgery Unit, Pancreas Center, "G.B. Rossi" University Hospital, Verona, Italy

Marina Paini Department of Surgery and Oncology, General Surgery Unit, Pancreas Center, "G.B. Rossi" University Hospital, Verona, Italy

Stefano Partelli Department of Surgery and Oncology, "G.B. Rossi" University Hospital, Verona, Italy and General Surgery Unit, "Sacro Cuore – Don Calabria" Hospital, Negrar (VR), Italy

Antonio Pea Department of Surgery and Oncology, General Surgery Unit, Pancreas Center, "G.B. Rossi" University Hospital, Verona, Italy

Paolo Pederzoli Department of Surgery and Oncology, General Surgery Unit, Pancreas Center, "G.B. Rossi" University Hospital, Verona, Italy

Federica Pedica Department of Pathology and Diagnostics, Pathology Unit, "G.B. Rossi" University Hospital, Verona, Italy

Silvia Pennacchio Department of Surgery and Oncology, General Surgery Unit, Pancreas Center, "G.B. Rossi" University Hospital, Verona, Italy

Roberto Pozzi Mucelli Department of Pathology and Diagnostics, Radiology Unit, "G.B. Rossi" University Hospital, Verona, Italy

Paolo Regi Surgery Unit, Casa di cura "Dr. P. Pederzoli", Peschiera del Garda (VR), Italy

Luigi Romano Radiology Unit, "Sacro Cuore - Don Calabria" Hospital, Negrar (VR), Italy

Roberto Salvia Department of Surgery and Oncology, General Surgery Unit, Pancreas Center, "G.B. Rossi" University Hospital, Verona, Italy

Aldo Scarpa Department of Pathology and Diagnostics, Pathology Unit, "G.B. Rossi" University Hospital and ARC-NET Research Centre, University of Verona, Verona, Italy

Marco Toaiari Department of Internal Medicine, "G.B. Rossi" University Hospital, Verona, Italy

Giampaolo Tortora Department of Medical Oncology, "G.B. Rossi" University Hospital, Verona, Italy

Chiara Trentin Department of Medical Oncology, "G.B. Rossi" University Hospital, Verona, Italy

Italo Vantini Department of Medicine, Pancreas Center, "G.B. Rossi" University Hospital, Verona, Italy

Duccio Volterrani Regional Center of Nuclear Medicine, University of Pisa Medical School, Pisa, Italy

Giuseppe Zamboni Department of Pathology and Diagnostics, "G.B. Rossi" University Hospital, Verona, Italy and Pathology Unit, "Sacro Cuore - Don Calabria" Hospital, Negrar (VR), Italy

Part I

Cystic Pancreatic Neoplasms

Roberto Salvia

Although considered uncommon, cystic neoplasms of the pancreas have been increasingly diagnosed due to the widespread use of cross-sectional imaging. In fact, in tertiary care centers with experience in pancreatic surgery, the proportion of pancreatic resections carried out for cystic neoplasms has doubled in the last two decades; in parallel, the number of patients enrolled in surveillance protocols has dramatically increased.

Pancreatic cystic neoplasms encompass a broad spectrum of benign, malignant, and borderline lesions. Many aspects of their biological behavior have been recently clarified, although an understanding of the natural history of mucinous forms—and especially of branch-duct intraductal papillary mucinous neoplasms (IPMNs)—is limited by the difficulty of distinguishing accurately between benign, malignant, and potentially malignant lesions before surgical resection. Furthermore, current guidelines for the management of pancreatic cystic neoplasms are based on the assumption that these lesions can be classified correctly on the basis of their cross-sectional imaging features. However, there is a certain degree of morphological overlap between different lesions such that the possibility of an inaccurate preoperative characterization must always be taken into account. Yet, some aspects of the management of pancreatic cystic neoplasms remain unclear, and, especially for mucinous neoplasms, the clinical and radiological work-up is not always able to predict the likelihood of progression to invasive cancer in a given patient. This has generated controversies as to whether patients should be offered resection or, alternatively, enrolled in surveillance protocols with periodic imaging. This is a relevant issue because these neoplasms are mostly diagnosed in asymptomatic patients who underwent cross-sectional imaging for unrelated problems.

R. Salvia (✉)
Department of Surgery and Oncology, General Surgery Unit, Pancreas Center,
"G.B. Rossi" University Hospital,
Verona, Italy
e-mail: roberto.salvia@ospedaleuniverona.it

P. Pederzoli and C. Bassi (eds.), *Uncommon Pancreatic Neoplasms*,
Updates in Surgery
DOI: 10.1007/978-88-470-2673-5_1, © Springer-Verlag Italia 2013

Among the many other unsettled aspects are the appropriate timeframe for surveillance, the role of cyst-fluid analysis and cytology, the role of atypical resections and of lymphadenectomy, and the recurrence rate of IPMNs and their association with other non-pancreatic neoplasms.

The diagnosis of pancreatic cystic neoplasms requires both a familiarity with the morphological spectrum of these lesions and the collaboration between surgeons, radiologists, gastroenterologists and pathologists, to increase the likelihood of appropriate management. At our institution, more than 6000 patients with pancreatic diseases presented between 1985 and 2011: 20% had cystic lesions. In the same period, more than 2200 pancreatic resections were carried out; of these, 23% were for cystic neoplasms. Thus, this section provides an overview of the current knowledge of pancreatic cystic neoplasms, with a particular focus on their more controversial aspects.

Another crucial aspect is the possibility to correctly predict the biological behavior of these lesions in order to ensure their proper clinical management.

The ability to detect genetic alterations in the cystic fluid, including the overexpression of oncogenes and the deletion of their suppressors, once routinely achievable, will likely provide us with the information we need to treat these patients.

This year the results of a consensus conference were published. Yet, as scientists we should remember that "expert opinions" form only the base of the pyramid of scientific evidence. With an increase in the number of clinical research projects and less reliance on consensus conferences we will be able to clarify the actual incidence, clinical behavior, and the best management of these uncommon (from a pathological point of view) diseases. Furthermore, our therapeutic experience must be communicated in order to accumulate evidence with the power of statistical significance.

Classification

1

Giuseppe Zamboni

Although cystic neoplasms of the pancreas were first reported in 1830, by Becourt [1], the classification of these lesions has become clearer only in the past three decades, following the work by Compagno and Oertel, who in 1978 divided these lesions in two different types: benign tumors with glycogen-rich cells, and mucinous cystic neoplasms with overt and latent malignancy [2]. The WHO classification of the exocrine tumors of the pancreas, published in 1996 [3], classified cystic neoplasms on the basis of the histopathological features of the cystic wall. The presence and characteristics of the epithelial lining allow pancreatic cystic neoplasm to be distinguished from other neoplastic non-epithelial lesions (lymphangioma, mixoid tumor, or leiomyoma), non-neoplastic epithelial lesions (lymphoepithelial cysts, retention cysts, enterogenous cysts, mucinous non-neoplastic cysts, unclassifiable cysts, ductal ectasia), non-neoplastic, non-epithelial lesions (pseudocysts), and other tissue alterations mimicking cystic neoplasms (chronic pancreatitis, fibrosis, autoimmune pancreatitis). The 2010 WHO histological classification of pancreatic cystic neoplasms is presented in Table 1.1 [4].

G. Zamboni (✉)
Department of Pathology and Diagnostics, "G.B. Rossi" University Hospital,
Verona, Italy and Pathology Unit, "Sacro Cuore - Don Calabria" Hospital,
Negrar (VR), Italy
e-mail: giuseppe.zamboni@sacrocuore.it

P. Pederzoli and C. Bassi (eds.), *Uncommon Pancreatic Neoplasms*,
Updates in Surgery
DOI: 10.1007/978-88-470-2673-5_1, © Springer-Verlag Italia 2013

Table 1.1 Histological classification of pancreatic cystic tumors (from [5])

Benign
Acinar cell cystadenoma
Serous cystadenoma

Premalignant lesions
Intraductal papillary mucinous neoplasms with low- or intermediate-grade dysplasia
Intraductal papillary mucinous neoplasms with high-grade dysplasia
Intraductal tubulopapillary neoplasms
Mucinous cystic neoplasms with low- or intermediate-grade dysplasia
Mucinous cystic neoplasms with high-grade dysplasia

Malignant
Acinar cell cystoadenocarcinoma
Intraductal papillary mucinous neoplasms with an associated invasive carcinoma
Mucinous cystic neoplasms with an associated invasive carcinoma
Serous cystoadenocarcinoma
Solid-pseudopapillary neoplasms

References

1. Becourt PJ BG (1830) Recherches sur le pancreas: ses fonctions et ses alterations organique. In: Strasbourg: FG Levrautl
2. Compagno J, Oertel JE (1978) Microcystic adenomas of the pancreas (glycogen-rich cystadenomas): a clinicopathologic study of 34 cases. Am J Clin Pathol 69:289-98
3. Compagno J, Oertel JE (1978) Mucinous cystic neoplasms of the pancreas with overt and latent malignancy (cystadenocarcinoma and cystadenoma). A clinicopathologic study of 41 cases. Am J Clin Pathol 69:573-80
4. Kloppel G SE, Longnecker DS, Capella C, Sobin LH (1996) Histogical typing of tumours of the esocrine pancreas. World Health Organization International Histological Classification of Tumours. Springer-Verlag, Berlin
5. Bosman FT, Carneiro F, Hruban RH et al (eds) (2010) World Health Organization classification of tumours of the digestive system, 4th edn. IARC, Lyon

Serous Cystic Neoplasms

2

Giuseppe Malleo, Giuseppe Zamboni, Marina Paini,
Giovanni Marchegiani and Riccardo Manfredi

2.1 Definition and Epidemiology

Serous cystic neoplasms (SCNs) are composed of non-atypical cuboidal, glycogen-rich, epithelial cells that produce a watery fluid. They are almost always benign lesions (serous cystadenomas), as only a very small number of malignant variants (serous cystoadenocarcinomas) has been described.

SCNs occur more frequently in middle-aged women. While any portion of the pancreatic gland can be affected, they are usually detected in the pancreatic head [1].

Five variants of SCN have been described: microcystic, macrocystic or oligocystic, mixed micro-macrocystic, von Hippel-Lindau (VHL)-associated, and solid. The majority of serous cystadenomas are microcystic, with a honeycomb-like appearance.

2.2 Serous Cystic Adenoma

2.2 1 Clinical Presentation

The majority of serous cystic adenomas (SCAs) are asymptomatic and thus incidentally discovered, typically on cross-sectional imaging performed for unrelated complaints. When present, the most common symptom is abdominal discomfort or low-grade pain. Weight loss, palpable mass, jaundice, and obstruction of the upper gastrointestinal tract are uncommon and may be

---

G. Malleo (✉)
Department of Surgery and Oncology, General Surgery Unit, Pancreas Center,
"G.B. Rossi" University Hospital,
Verona, Italy
e-mail: giuseppe.malleo@ospedaleuniverona.it

P. Pederzoli and C. Bassi (eds.), *Uncommon Pancreatic Neoplasms*,
Updates in Surgery
DOI: 10.1007/978-88-470-2673-5_2, © Springer-Verlag Italia 2013

ascribed to a mass effect on surrounding organs. A correct clinical and radiological diagnosis is of paramount importance because this neoplasm, unlike other cystic neoplasms of the pancreas, is almost always benign. Whenever possible, a conservative approach is considered to be the treatment of choice.

Although symptoms may not be helpful for diagnostic purposes, they can grossly indicate a benign or malignant neoplasm. The diagnosis of SCA should also be considered in the presence of von Hippel-Lindau (VHL) syndrome, which is a genetic condition that in 15–30% of cases is associated with cystic lesions, including SCA [2, 3].

2.2.2 Diagnostic Imaging

Ultrasound (US) is usually the first step in the diagnostic work up of patients with suspected SCAs. In fact, due to its widespread use in clinical practice, US has significantly increased the number of incidental SCA observations. The diagnosis is easily made when sonography shows a mass with lobulated margins, no posterior acoustic enhancement, and an internal honeycomb-like architecture, due to the presence of multiple septa delimiting small (< 2 cm diameter) cystic spaces (Fig. 2.1). In 10–30% of cases, calcifications within the septa are seen, and even less frequently a central calcified scar [4]. The microcystic appearance is also typical of SCA associated with VHL syndrome but in these cases the lesion is multicentric or diffusely involves the whole

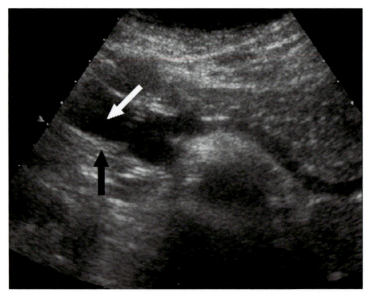

Fig. 2.1 Serous cystadenoma: ultrasound (US). Sonographic scans show a hypoechoic lesion with sharp margins in the head of the pancreas (*black arrow*). Within the lesion, anechoic areas can be observed, corresponding to the cystic spaces (*white arrow*)

gland. There are two reasons why US may fail to recognize the microcystic pattern of SCA: (1) in the presence of a sponge-like mass in which the multiplicity of the small cysts and the thick fibrous stroma produce the false impression that the tumor is solid, and (2) in cases of mixed tumors, when the macrocystic component conceals the microcystic one, resulting in the misdiagnosis of a macrocystic mass. The macrocystic type is easily detectable even when the tumor is small. The appearance is that of a sharply marginated, hypoechoic mass; however, if there are sparse, thin central septa the differential diagnosis from other cystic masses is very difficult. In mixed SCAs, together with the microcysts, larger (> 2 cm) cystic spaces can be found at the periphery of the lesion, resulting in a mixed pattern. The macrocyst can enlarge up to 8–10 cm, such that recognition of the true nature of the tumor becomes difficult. The false-negative rate is low and is due to tumor location (tail) or patient characteristics (obesity, meteorism).

The computed tomography (CT) appearance of SCA depends on the macroscopic feature of the tumor and on the timing of data acquisition. Microcystic tumors are seen as an unenhanced mass, sometimes deforming the profile of the gland, when peripherally located. The density is homogeneous and may be the same or slightly superior to that of water but more frequently hypodense compared to adjacent pancreatic parenchyma (Fig. 2.2). Calcifications may occur in 30% of the cases; when present, they are centrally located (Fig. 2.2) and punctate or globular, as opposed to the lamellar calcifications seen in mucinous cystic tumors [5]. A central fibrous scar is visible in 47% of the

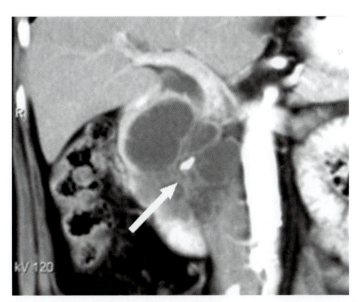

Fig. 2.2 Serous cystadenoma: Coronal multiplanar reconstructed, contrast-enhanced CT shows a multicystic, microcyst focal pancreatic lesion in the head of the pancreas. The lesion shows a central scar and a central calcification (*arrow*)

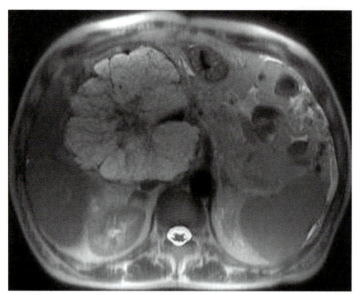

Fig. 2.3 Serous cystadenoma: Axial T2-weighted MRI shows a serous cystadenoma of the head of the pancreas. The neoplasm shows the multicystic, microcystic features responsible for the "honeycomb" pattern

cases, especially in larger masses since it forms later in tumor development (Fig. 2.2). Maximal visualization of the septa is possible on contrast-enhanced CT in the pancreatic parenchymal phase as well as based on the honeycomb appearance. A cystic mass with a central calcification in conjunction with a central scar is highly indicative of SCA. In the mixed forms, peripheral macrocysts are even more easily recognizable on CT than by US, making the diagnosis easier. In the delayed phase of contrast enhancement, septal recognition is very difficult due to the intracystic liquid. Macrocystic patterns are indistinguishable from other macrocystic masses of the pancreas, such as mucinous cystic tumors.

Magnetic resonance imaging (MRI) is increasingly assuming a major role in the work up of these patients due to its capability to simultaneously assess the pancreatic parenchyma and the pancreatic ductal system. In the microcystic pattern of SCA, even a small content of fluid within the dense septa of a "sponge-like" mass can be seen on MRI; however, this technique has the disadvantage that it is insensitive to calcifications [6] (Fig. 2.3). In macro-microcystic forms, the two components are well recognizable. An even better evaluation of the spatial relation between the mass and the biliary or pancreatic duct is obtained with magnetic resonance cholangiopancreatography (MRCP), which distinguishes these tumors from intraductal papillary mucinous neoplasms (IPMNs), particularly when the tumor is located in the head or the uncinate process of the gland. MRCP should be routinely carried out in the staging of these tumors since it helps to distinguish microcystic SCA from intraductal tumors of the peripheral branches, with their septate appearance [7]. The presence/absence of communication with the pancreatic duct system is diagnostic and is useful for the differential diagnosis between SCA and IPMN.

In the oligocystic forms of SCA, the MRI aspects are non-specific and do not lead to a definitive differential diagnosis from mucinous forms.

2.2.3 Pathology

Serous cystadenomas frequently present as a well-circumscribed, round, cystic masses ranging from 1 to 25 cm in their greatest dimension, depending on whether the lesions are symptomatic (large lesions) or an incidental finding. SCAs show no communication with the pancreatic ducts. Macroscopically, they are subdivided into five subtypes according to the number, dimensions, and distribution of the individual lobules:

1. Microcystic or classic type: The relatively well circumscribed neoplasm features bosselated margins. On sectioning, these lesions are sponge-like, formed by innumerable cysts that range in diameter from 1 to 5 mm, with only few larger (up to 1–2 cm) cysts, frequently peripherally located. The cysts are filled with clear, watery fluid. Typically, this type presents with a central stellate scar that frequently shows calcium deposits. These deposits are the pathological basis of the typical "sunburst" pattern of calcification seen on radiological studies (Fig 2.4a);
2. Macrocystic or oligocystic type: These neoplasms are characterized by a small number of locules and are less well-demarcated than the microcystic variant, due to extension of the cysts into the adjacent pancreatic parenchyma. The fluids contained in the cysts may vary from the classic clear and watery to bloody and brown. The cut surface shows the presence of a distinct number of cysts (oligocystic) or sometimes a single cyst (unilocular) > 2 cm in diameter, even reaching 10–15 cm (Fig 2.4b). In this form, the central scar is characteristically lacking such that these tumors usually present as an ill-defined growth;
3. Mixed micro-macrocystic type: In this form, a mixture of micro- and macro-locules is typically present, sometimes with a central scar;
4. Solid type: In a minority of cases, there is a pure solid growth lacking either cystic locules or a central scar. These are usually small lesions, measuring 2–4 cm in their greatest dimension, and comprising small acini lined by the typical serous cells;
5. Serous cystic neoplasms associated with VHL syndrome: This form is characterized by multiple, mixed type, serous adenomas that may partly or diffusely involve the entire pancreas. The epithelial serous cells are virtually indistinguishable from those occurring sporadically.

Microscopically, the five subtypes are indistinguishable from one another,

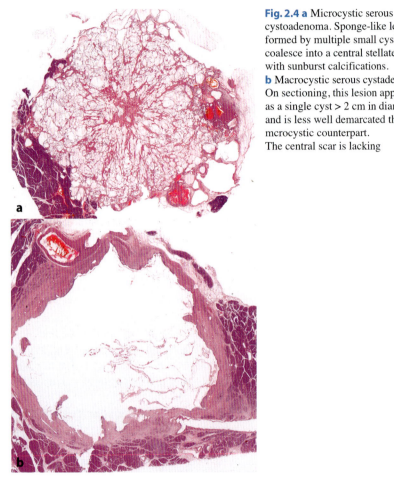

Fig. 2.4 a Microcystic serous cystoadenoma. Sponge-like lesion formed by multiple small cysts that coalesce into a central stellate scar with sunburst calcifications.
b Macrocystic serous cystadenoma. On sectioning, this lesion appears as a single cyst > 2 cm in diameter, and is less well demarcated than the mcrocystic counterpart. The central scar is lacking

as they exhibit a typical cuboidal to almost flat serous epithelium. The cells are characterized by a clear cytoplasm and round nuclei, with inconspicuous nucleoli. Neither cytological atypia nor mitotic activity are seen. Intracellular glycogen is characteristic (deposits positive for periodic-acid–Schiff, diastase-sensitive) (Fig 2.5). The neoplastic stroma is highly vascular, creating a fine supporting network. The septa separating the larger cysts are hyalinized and contain hemosiderin-laden macrophages, sometimes with entrapped islets of Langerhans and exocrine acini.

Immunohistochemically, the epithelium shows positivity for low molecular weight cytokeratins (CK 7, 8, 18, and 19), diffuse membrane staining for EMA, and focal staining for CA 19-9. Serous cystic neoplasms associated with VHL syndrome show a dysregulation of the VHL/HIF (hypoxia-inducible factor) pathway, with the expression of HIF-1α.

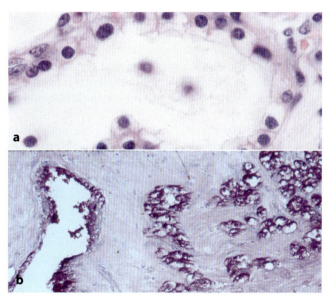

Fig. 2.5 Serous cystadenoma. Typical histologic appearance of epithelial lining, consisting of cuboidal cells with clear cytoplasm (**a**), glycogen-filled, and PAS-positive (**b**)

The finding of a mass in the pancreatic head with the above-mentioned features in a female patient without dilation of the main pancreatic duct, a normal parenchyma, and calcifications leads to the diagnosis of SCN. The diagnosis can be considered definitive when the lesion shows a mixed aspect, with macrocysts in the periphery of a microcystic core. Despite the microcystic aspect, when in a male patient the cystic mass is located in the uncinate process and associated with a main duct dilation, the diagnosis is more difficult. In these cases, the differential diagnosis will include a branch-duct IPMN, such that it is mandatory to demonstrate a relationship between the mass and the main pancreatic duct. MRCP is useful for this purpose, but when the lesion is very close to the main duct endoscopic retrograde cholangiopancreatography may be necessary. As previously noted, SCNs can appear as solid lesions, leading to a misdiagnosis with other brightly enhancing solid lesions, such as non-functioning neuroendocrine tumors. In these cases, MRI will be able to detect the microcystic aspect and a peripheral wall.

Macrocystic SCNs lack proper radiological characterization on US, CT, and MRI; instead, endoscopic US seems to be the only technique able to supply further information. Analysis of the cyst fluid for CEA helps in differentiating mucinous from serous cysts, as in the former values are usually > 192 ng/ml (sensitivity 75% and specificity 84%, accuracy 79%). CEA values < 5 ng/ml predict a benign cyst (sensitivity 54%, positive predictive value 94%) [8].

2.2.4 Treatment

Resection is generally carried out in symptomatic patients with very large SCAs or when the tumor cannot be distinguished from other cystic tumors of the pancreas (mucinous cystadenoma, IPMN). Some authors recommend resection for all SCAs but we believe that a more selective approach should be considered.

In a report by Tseng et al. [9], 106 patients with SCNs were analyzed to better define the natural history of the disease and its optimal management. In that series, 47% of the patients were asymptomatic while among those with symptoms abdominal pain was the most common. The large lesions (> 4 cm) were significantly associated with the presence of symptoms. In 24 patients, serial radiography was available and analyzed; the median growth rate was 0.6 cm/year, but in tumors > 4 cm it was 1.98 cm/year [9].

However, a recent study from our institution of 145 patients with SCN enrolled in a surveillance protocol with serial MRI + MRCP showed that the overall mean growth rate was only 0.28 cm/year. There were two distinct phases of growth during follow-up: 0.1 cm/year during the first 7 years and 0.6 cm/year thereafter. The oligocystic/macrocystic variant, a history of other non-pancreatic malignancies, and patient age were demonstrated to impact tumor growth. Tumor size at the time of diagnosis was not a predictor of growth and therefore should not be used for decisional purposes. A surveillance protocol with MRI + MRCP can be proposed for all patients with well characterized and asymptomatic SCN, but those with factors that impact tumor growth should be informed of the increased likelihood of a pancreatic resection in the long-term. A follow-up time frame of 2 years seems to be appropriate [10].

2.3 Serous Cystoadenocarcinoma

Although SCNs are considered as benign in virtually all cases, serous cystoadenocarcinomas have been described, none of them at our institution. To date, about 25 cases have been reported in the literature, implying a risk of malignancy of around 3% [11]. Patients with cystoadenocarcinoma were between 52 and 81 years of age; two-thirds were women [5] and most were asymptomatic.

References

1. Bassi C, Salvia R, Molinari E et al (2003) Management of 100 consecutive cases of pancreatic serous cystadenoma: wait for symptoms and see at imaging or vice versa? World J Surg 27:319-323
2. Neumann HP, Dinkel E, Brambs H et al (1991) Pancreatic lesions in the von Hippel-Lindau syndrome. Gastroenterology 101:465-471

3. Girelli R, Bassi C, Falconi M et al (1997) Pancreatic cystic manifestations in von Hippel-Lindau disease. Int J Pancreatol 22:101-109
4. Procacci C, Graziani R, Bicego E et al (1997) Serous cystadenoma of the pancreas: report of 30 cases with emphasis on the imaging findings. J Comput Assist Tomogr 21:373-382
5. Procacci C, Biasiutti C, Carbognin G et al (1999) Characterization of cystic tumors of the pancreas: CT accuracy. J Comput Assist Tomogr 23:906-912
6. Nishihara K, Kawabata A, Ueno T et al (1996) The differential diagnosis of pancreatic cysts by MR imaging. Hepatogastroenterology 43:714-720
7. Carbognin G (2003) Serous cystic tumors. Springer-Verlag, New York
8. Van der Waaij LA, Delleman HM, Porte RJ (2005) Cyst fluid analysis in the differential diagnosis of pancreatic cystic lesions: a pooled analysis. Gastrointest Endosc 62:383-389
9. Tseng JF, Warshaw AL, Sahani DV et al (2005) Serous cystadenoma of the pancreas: tumor growth rates and recommendations for treatment. Ann Surg 242:413-419
10: Malleo G, Bassi C, Rossini R et al (2012) Growth pattern of serous cystic neoplasms of the pancreas: observational study with long-term magnetic resonance surveillance and recommendations for treatment. Gut 61:746-751
11. Strobel O, Z'Graggen K, Schmitz-Winnenthal FH et al (2003) Risk of malignancy in serous cystic neoplasms of the pancreas. Digestion 68:24-33

Mucinous Cystic Neoplasms

3

Giovanni Marchegiani, Riccardo Manfredi,
Giuseppe Malleo, Isabella Frigerio and Giuseppe Zamboni

3.1 Definition and Epidemiology

Mucinous cystic neoplasms (MCNs) are pancreatic cystic epithelial neoplasms occurring almost exclusively in women. They are formed by epithelial cells producing mucin and supported by an ovarian-type stroma, without communication with the pancreatic ductal system. According to the grade of epithelial dysplasia, these tumors are classified as MCN with low-grade dysplasia, moderate dysplasia, or high-grade dysplasia (carcinoma in situ). If there is an invasive carcinoma component, the lesions are designated MCN with associated invasive carcinoma [1].

MCNs are preferentially located in the body and tail of the pancreas. The patient age at presentation range is broad, with an average that seems to depend on the degree of malignancy of the neoplasm. Thus, patients with malignant MCN are typically older, suggesting a time-related degeneration of the tumor from an initially benign lesion. The incidence of malignancy for MCN is 17.5%, as reported in the MGH-Verona series [2]. An early diagnosis of MCN is essential since the prognosis for patients with the malignant form is the same as for those with ductal adenocarcinoma, while for patients with "in situ" MCNs surgery could be curative.

At best, MCN is a pre-malignant lesion and it is therefore important to distinguish it from other cystic lesions of the pancreas. On pathological examination, the same tumor may simultaneously exhibit all the various degrees of malignant transformation. This is of great pathogenic relevance as it suggests an adenoma-carcinoma sequence [3].

G. Marchegiani (✉)
Department of Surgery and Oncology, General Surgery Unit, Pancreas Center,
"G.B. Rossi" University Hospital,
Verona, Italy
e-mail: giuseppe.marchegiani@ospedaleuniverona.it

P. Pederzoli and C. Bassi (eds.), *Uncommon Pancreatic Neoplasms*,
Updates in Surgery
DOI: 10.1007/978-88-470-2673-5_3, © Springer-Verlag Italia 2013

3.2 Clinical Findings

The symptoms in MCNs are non-specific and are not particularly helpful in the differential diagnosis of pancreatic cystic lesions. The most frequent symptoms are abdominal discomfort or pain. Uncommonly, the patient complains of abdominal pain located in the upper quadrants that irradiates to the flanks, which could guide a pancreatic localization. However, there may also be non-specific symptoms suggestive of malignancy, such as weight loss, anorexia, and obstructive jaundice.

3.3 Diagnostic Imaging

Two patterns of MCN are seen on diagnostic imaging procedures: *macrocystic multilocular* and *macrocystic unilocular* [4]. While not pathognomonic, the former is frequently located in the body-tail of the gland. On ultrasound (US) images, macrocystic multilocular forms appear as a sharply defined mass surrounded by a variably thickened wall (Fig. 3.1). Thin septae delimit the cystic spaces, and calcifications are a common finding. On computed tomography (CT) scan, the pre-contrast phase can easily reveal calcifications. The density of the content of these tumors depends on the amount of mucin or the fluid-fluid level from underlying bleeding. This pattern is clearly demonstrated by contrast medium, as the walls and septae are of lower enhancement than the surrounding pancreatic parenchyma because of the fibrous tissue composition

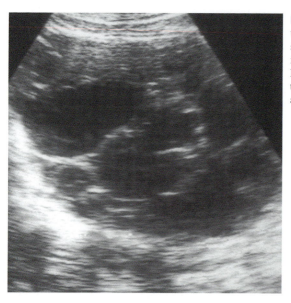

Fig. 3.1 Mucinous cystedenoma ultrasound. The sonographic scan shows a hypoechoic lesion in the head of the pancreas. The lesions has a macrocystic pattern, as indicated by the large anechoic central areas

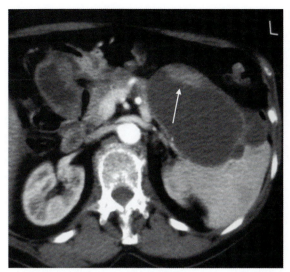

Fig. 3.2 Mucinous cystedenoma. Axial contrast-enhanced computed tomography scan shows a oligocystic-macrocystic lesion in the body-tail of the pancreas. The cystic lesion contains a mural nodule on the non-dependent wall of the lesion (*arrow*)

and minimal vascularization. The outer wall and septae are of similar thickness. The macrocystic unilocular pattern is less specific and may simulate any other pancreatic cystic mass, at US and at CT. Consequently, in cases with unique cysts with a thin wall, no calcifications, and no parietal nodules the diagnosis is not easily made.

From the radiological point of view, a thickened wall, the presence of papillary projections arising from the wall or septae, evidence of peripheral calcifications, and invasion of the surrounding vascular structures are considered the best signs of malignancy (Fig. 3.2). The diagnosis will be clearer if extracapsular extension of the lesion is detected on CT contrast-enhanced images. When thick walls, thick septae, and calcifications are simultaneously present, the probability of malignancy is 95%. When fewer than three signs are present, the probability of malignancy decreases, and it is zero when there are no calcifications and the septae and the wall are thin. Since calcifications cannot be detected by magnetic resonance imaging (MRI), the primary imaging modality for these patients is CT.

The predominant fluid content of MCNs renders them brighter on T2-weighted MRI, which well depicts the presence, features, and distribution of the internal septae. Magnetic resonance cholangiopancreatography (MRCP) is optimal for the non-invasive assessment of the pancreatic duct system (Wirsung and Santorini ducts) (Fig. 3.3). When the mass is clearly isolated from the ductal system, thereby excluding the possibility of an intraductal tumor, further examination with MRCP is not required (Fig. 3.3).

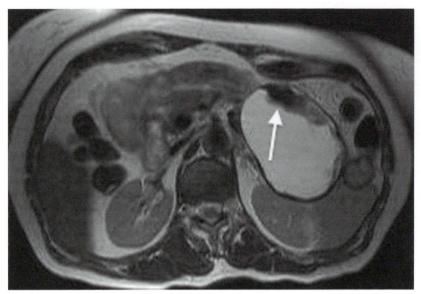

Fig. 3.3 Mucinous cystedenoma. Axial T2-weighted magnetic resonance image shows a cystic macrocystic lesion in the body-tail of the pancreas, with hypointense mural nodules on the non-dependent wall of the lesion (*arrow*)

3.4 Pathology

The overwhelming majority of MCNs occur in the body-tail of the pancreas, where the tumor presents as a round mass with a smooth surface and a fibrous pseudocapsule of variable thickness and frequently containing calcifications. The size of these neoplasms in their greatest dimension ranges from 2 to 35 cm, with an average of 6–10 cm. The cut section shows either a unilocular or a multilocular tumor with cystic spaces ranging in diameter from a few millimeters to several centimeters and containing either thick mucin or a mixture of mucin and hemorrhagic-necrotic material. The internal surface of unilocular tumors is usually smooth and glistening, whereas multilocular tumors often show papillary projections and mural nodules. There is no significant size difference among the different MCN categories, whereas the malignancy of the tumor correlates significantly with the presence of papillary projections and/or mural nodules and multilocularity. As noted above, the tumor does not communicate with the duct of Wirsung or the secondary ducts.

Microscopically, MCNs show two distinct components: an inner epithelial layer and an outer densely cellular "ovarian-like" stromal layer (Fig. 3.4). The mucin-producing epithelium exhibits a spectrum of differentiation, ranging from histologically benign appearing columnar epithelium to severely atypical epithelium.

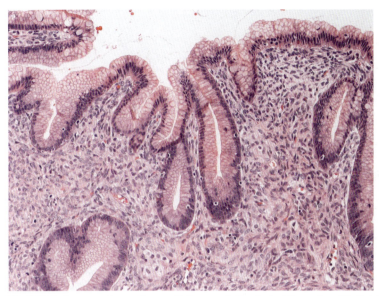

Fig. 3.4 Mucinous cystic neoplasm with low-grade dysplasia. The cyst wall is lined with a mildly dysplastic columnar epithelium supported by an "ovarian-like" stroma

The recent World Health Organization (WHO 2010) classification of MCNs [5] comprises the three above-mentioned types: MCN with low-grade dysplasia, with moderate-grade epithelial dysplasia; and with high-grade dysplasia, characterized by severe dysplasia-carcinoma in situ changes (Fig. 3.5). The presence of carcinomatous stromal invasion defines MCNs with associated invasive carcinoma. The invasive component usually resembles the common ductal adenocarcinoma.

Immunophenotypically, the mucinous epithelial cells show immunoreactivity with epithelial markers, including EMA, CEA, cytokeratins 7, 8, 18, and 19, and MUC5AC, a gastric-type marker of mucin. Focally, there is positivity for intestinal type mucins (MUC2) in goblet cells scattered within the epithelium. The invasive component is frequently positive for MUC1 and p53. The ovarian-like stroma is positive for vimentin, smooth-muscle actin, and progesterone receptors (Fig. 3.6a), while the luteinized epithelioid cells stain for α-inhibin (Fig. 3.6b).

3.5 Differential Diagnosis

The macrocystic multilocular pattern is considered typical but it is not pathognomonic. Oligocystic serous cystic neoplasms (SCNs), solid pseudopapillary tumors (cystic variant), and cystic endocrine tumors are identical in appear-

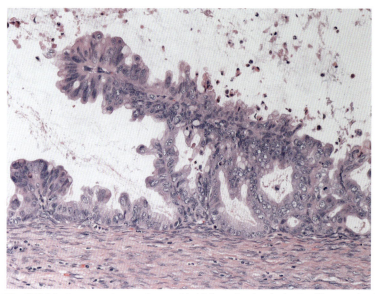

Fig. 3.5 Mucinous cystic neoplasm with high-grade dysplasia. Papillary projections lined by severe dysplastic epithelium

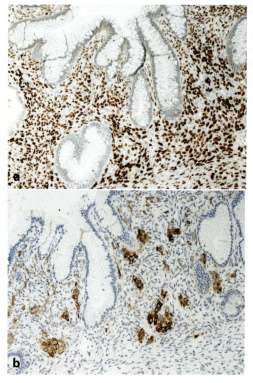

Fig. 3.6 Mucinous cystic neoplasm. The ovarian-like stroma shows nuclear positivity for progesterone receptors (**a**) and α-inhibin cytoplasmic positivity in the luteinized cells (**b**)

ance to MCNs. In these cases, clinical history and laboratory data are essential for the correct diagnosis. Oligocystic SCN can almost never be pre-operatively differentiated from benign MCN.

In neuroendocrine and pseudopapillary tumors, the cystic component is due to previous necrosis and intratumoral bleeding. In the former, the clinical syndrome might suggest the diagnosis; in the latter, MRI will enhance the differences in the appearance of the fluid content.

Pseudocysts make the diagnosis challenging, as they can resemble the macrocystic unilocular pattern of MCN. If the clinical history is silent, MCN should be suspected.

3.6 Treatment

When possible, all MCNs should be resected, both cystadenomas and cystadenocarcinomas. Current thinking is that all MCNs have the potential to progress to malignancy. Given the life-expectancy of most of these patients, almost always middle-aged women, there is a high risk of development of mucinous cystadenocarcinoma, which, unfortunately, has a very low rate of resectability and a very poor prognosis. Predictors of malignancy are: large size (≥ 4 cm) and the presence of nodules, septae, and "eggshell" calcifications. In these cases, surgical "standard" pancreatic resection should be performed, avoiding middle pancreatectomies and spleen-preserving distal pancreatectomies [6, 7].

References

1. Zamboni G, Scarpa A, Bogina G et al (1999) Mucinous cystic tumors of the pancreas: clinicopathological features, prognosis, and relationship to other mucinous cystic tumors. Am J Surg Pathol 23:410-422
2. Crippa S, Salvia R,Warshaw AL et al (2008) Mucinous cystic neoplasm of the pancreas is not an aggressive entity: lessons from 163 resected patients. Ann Surg 247:571c9
3. Furukawa T, Takahashi T, Kobari M et al (1992) The mucus-hypersecreting tumor of the pancreas. Development and extension visualized by three-dimensional computerized mapping. Cancer 70:1505-1513
4. Sperti C, Cappellazzo F, Pasquali C et al (1993) Cystic neoplasms of the pancreas: problems in differential diagnosis. Am Surg 59:740-745
5. Koito K, Namieno T, Ichimura T et al (1998) Mucin-producing pancreatic tumors: comparison of MR cholangiopancreatography with endoscopic retrograde cholangiopancreatography. Radiology 208:231-237
6. Tanaka M, Chari S,Adsay V et al (2005) International consensus guidelines for management of intraductal papillary mucinous neoplasms and mucinous cystic neoplasms of the pancreas. Pancreatology 6:17-32
7. Baleur YL, Couvelard A, Vullierme MP et al (2011) Mucinous cystic neoplasms of the pancreas: definition of preoperative imaging criteria for high-risk lesions. Pancreatology11:495-499

Solid-pseudopapillary, Acinar, and Other Cystic Neoplasms

4

Marina Paini, Giuseppe Zamboni, Riccardo Manfredi, Salvatore Paiella and Giuseppe Malleo

4.1 Solid Papillary Neoplasms

4.1.1 Definition and Epidemiology

Solid papillary neoplasms (SPNs) are a low-grade malignant neoplasm occurring predominantly in young women. The tumors are composed of poorly cohesive, monomorphic epithelial cells forming solid and pseudopapillary structures that frequently undergo hemorrhagic-cystic degeneration (WHO 2010).

Among the cystic neoplasms, SPNs of the pancreas are the least common. They were reported for the first time in 1959 by Franz [1]. Since then, this tumor has been described under different names: solid tumor, cystic-solid, papillary-epithelial, and cystic papillary. In the last few years, the number of literature reports of patients with SPNs has increased, owing to the improved recognition of these lesions.

SPN is a slow-growing, low-aggressive tumor, and even when malignant usually has a favorable prognosis [2]. However, 10–15% of all patients have metastases, which are frequently present at the time of first diagnosis [3]. From an epidemiological point of view, most (> 90%) of the patients with SPNs are young females, between 30 and 40 years of age. The relationship between tumor development and risk factors is not yet known.

M. Paini (✉)
Department of Surgery and Oncology, General Surgery Unit, Pancreas Center,
"G.B. Rossi" University Hospital,
Verona, Italy
e-mail: marinapaini@gmail.com.it

P. Pederzoli and C. Bassi (eds.), *Uncommon Pancreatic Neoplasms*,
Updates in Surgery
DOI: 10.1007/978-88-470-2673-5_4, © Springer-Verlag Italia 2013

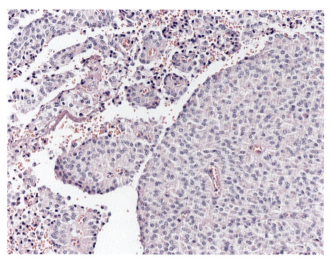

Fig. 4.1 Solid-pseudopapillary neoplasm. Pseudopapillary structures with fibrovascular cores (*left*) and a solid area showing small monomorphic cells (*right*)

4.1.2 Pathology

Macroscopically, SPNs are typically large, round, well-circumscribed masses that exhibit variable proportions of solid and cystic areas filled with hemorrhagic fluid and necrotic debris. Regarding their macroscopic appearances, at the extreme ends of the spectrum are the exclusively solid SPNs (usually the smaller lesions) and the entirely cystic SPNs (usually the larger tumors). The latter may be easily mistaken for a pseudocyst.

Microscopically, the tumors are composed of a mixture of solid and cystic areas, often surrounded by a fibrous capsule. The tumor cells, both in solid areas and lining the pseudopapillae, are monomorphous, with round to oval nuclei and an eosinophilic, granular cytoplasm (Fig. 4.1). PAS-positive globules, stromal myxoid degeneration, necrotic changes with foam cells, and hemorrhage are characteristically present. Mitotic figures are virtually absent, consistent with the low proliferative fraction (Ki-67 index < 2%). Pathologically, the most important differential diagnosis included with SPNs is endocrine neoplasms. The immunophenotype may help to distinguish the two, as SPNs are positive for CD10, vimentin, and nuclear β-catenin (Fig. 4.2). Progesterone receptor (PR) positivity supports the hypothesis of their pathogenetic role.

SPN should be regarded as a carcinoma of low malignant potential and a favorable clinical course, although both the invasion of vital structures and metastases have been reported [4-8]. Over 95% of patients with SPNs limited to the pancreas are cured by complete surgical resection. Only a few patients die of metastasizing tumor [9-11].

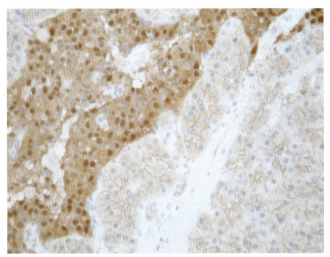

Fig. 4.2 Solid-pseudopapillary neoplasm. Cytoplasmic and nuclear β-catenin immunostaining in neoplastic cells (*left*); a weak membranous positivity is seen in normal pancreas (*right*)

4.1.3 Clinical Findings

Abdominal pain is the predominant and, sometimes, the only symptom present. The pain may be associated with a palpable abdominal mass, anorexia, or weight loss, but any of these signs may occur in isolation. The appearance of an abdominal mass is not considered to be a symptom. Rather, these patients usually complain of a full sensation and abdominal discomfort, and only on examination can a mass be appreciated, especially in the left upper quadrant. The simultaneous presence of pain and an abdominal mass does not suffice to confirm the pancreatic origin of the lesion.

The non-specific clinical features and the young mean age at the time of presentation are frequent reasons for the tendency to underestimate this tumor, by patients and doctors. For the latter, it could be useful to divide these patients based on the anatomical location of the lesion. In our experience, abdominal pain is more often present when the tumor is located in the body-tail of the pancreas, and in some cases is related to weight loss and abdominal discomfort, when a mean tumor diameter of 8.8 cm is reached. Fewer symptoms occur with tumors with a mean diameter of 5.4 cm and located in the head of the pancreas; in such cases, jaundice is seen in 4% of patients and gastrointestinal discomfort in 8%. Thus, it can be assumed that symptoms, in particular abdominal pain, are related to the size and behavior of the tumor, which involves near-by structures. This is different from the abdominal pain associated with ductal carcinoma of the pancreas, which is due to retroperitoneal nerve infiltration. The difference between the sizes and symptoms of SPNs are probably due to their slow evolution and low grade of malignancy.

4.1.4 Laboratory Findings

Laboratory data are not significant in these tumors due to the lack of a specific tumor marker. Chromogranin A, which has a higher sensitivity for endocrine tumors (68%), could be useful in the differential diagnosis between non-functioning endocrine neoplasms and SPNs [12], although the literature reports a positive result in the absence of an endocrine tumor in 19% of cases [13]. In our experience, the chromogranin A test was always negative in SPNs.

4.1.5 Diagnostic Imaging

Solid papillary neoplasms are well-vascularized and encapsulated masses with definite margins [14] (Fig. 4.3). Calcifications and septa may be seen inside the mass but they are not pathognomonic. Instead, the distinctive findings of these tumors are the alternation of solid and cystic areas, in which a necrotic hemorrhagic component may be present [15] (Fig. 4.4a, b). These findings may be seen in the same lesion, possibly with differences in the proportions of the two components.

The lesions are sometimes reported as cystic even though the finding of a rich vascularization could lead to their being mistaken for neuroendocrine tumors.

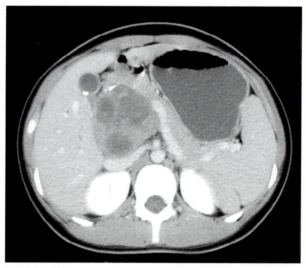

Fig. 4.3 Solid pseudopapillary neoplasm (SPN). Axial contrast-enhanced computed tomography shows a solid pseudopapillary neoplasm in the head of the pancreas that appears hypodense, with an heterogeneous pattern

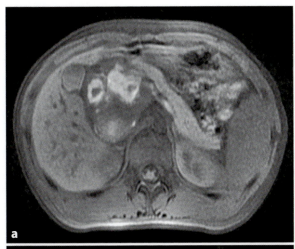
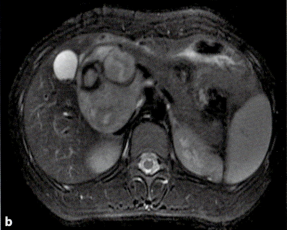

Fig. 4.4 Solid pseudopapillary neoplasm (SPN). **a** Axial fat-saturated T1-weighted magnetic resonance image shows hypointense solid pseudopapillary neoplasm in the head of the pancreas. The internal areas of the neoplasm are hyperintense on T1-weighted images, suggestive of the presence of methemoglobin. **b** On the axial fat-saturated T2-weighted image, the solid pseudopapillary neoplasm appears hyperintense, with an heterogeneous pattern

4.1.6 Treatment

Surgical treatment must be considered in all the patients diagnosed with SPNs, based on the still unknown biological behavior and potential malignancy of these tumors. The laparoscopic approach has been shown to be safe and feasible, if expertise is available; the median follow-up is 47 months (range 5–98). Care must be taken during surgery to prevent specimen rupture [16]. Metastatic disease is not considered a contraindication to surgery, as survival after the resection of liver metastases exceeds 5 years (range 6 months to 17 years). Recurrences are seen mainly in malignant SPNs but the long-term survival of these patients has been reported if they are treated [17-19].

4.2 Acinar Cell Cystadenoma, Cystadenocarcinoma, and Other Cystic Neoplasms

4.2.1 Acinar Cell Cystadenoma

Acinar cell cystadenoma (ACA) is a benign cystic lesion lined by cells with cytological features of acinar differentiation and evidence of pancreatic exocrine enzyme production [20]. ACAs show no clear age predilection; with patients ranging in age from 16 to 66 years, but there is a female predominance.

ACAs can be divided into two categories: clinically recognized macroscopic lesions and incidental microscopic findings. Macroscopically, the former are well circumscribed, cystic lesions with a thin, fibrous pseudocapsule that in some cases can instead be thick and contain calcifications. Microscopically, the cysts are lined by a single layer of cuboidal or columnar cells, with little tendency to pseudostratification or crowding, and with the typical features of acinar cells, i.e., cytoplasmic eosinophilic granules and immunoreactivity for the acinar marker trypsin (Fig. 4.5a, b). Thus, ACAs are thought represent the benign counterpart of the well-recognized acinar cell cystadenocarcinoma [21-24].

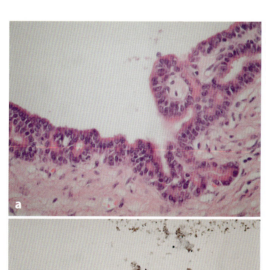

Fig. 4.5 Acinar cell cystadenoma. **a** Cyst lined by columnar cells (H&E staining). **b** Immunohistochemical expression of the acinar differentiation marker trypsin

4.2.2 Acinar Cell Cystadenocarcinoma

Rare examples of cystic acinar cell carcinoma have been reported as "acinar cell cystadenocarcinomas" [22, 25]. In contrast to ACAs, the patients are frequently men, with a mean age of 50–60 years. Macroscopically, these neoplasms are large masses, with diameters up to 35 cm, that contain multiple cysts, with a diameter ranging from a few millimeters to several centimeters. Hemorrhage and necrosis have been reported [26]. Microscopically, the multiple cysts, are admixed with tubular and solid areas. The lining cells show the typical acinar differentiation, with a cytoplasm filled with deeply eosinophilic granules in the apex and basophilic staining at the base. The cells composing cystic acinar cell carcinomas showed clear signs of atypia, with many mitoses; areas of necrosis are frequently present as well.

The prognosis of these patients, as reported in the literature, is similar to that of patients with the solid counterpart of these tumors. Most patients present with metastatic disease, either at the time of diagnosis or a few months post-operatively.

4.2.3 Other Cystic Neoplasms

This category includes very rare lesions, which account for less than 5% of cystic neoplasms.

Cystic endocrine neoplasms are characterized by solid growth, with massive degenerative changes. They may be confused with other cystic neoplasms but the preoperative diagnosis can be obtained with fine-needle aspiration biopsy, which reveals the characteristic cytology [27, 28]. The diagnosis may be confirmed by the immunohistochemical demonstration of endocrine markers, such as chromogranin A and synaptophysin, and of hormone production [29].

Lymphoepithelial cysts are benign, uncommon lesions characterized by mature squamous epithelium associated with lymphoid tissue [30]. They are more common in men, with a mean patient age of 56 years. Macroscopically, they may occur predominantly as extrapancreatic lesions and in any case are well demarcated from the surrounding pancreatic parenchyma. They are either multilocular (60% of cases) or unilocular (40% of cases), and their mean dimension is 4.7 cm. The cyst wall is usually thin and the inner surface of the cysts is smooth or finely granular. Microscopically, the lining epithelium of the cysts is stratified squamous epithelium, admixed with flat or cuboidal epithelium. The cyst wall and the septae are filled with dense lymphoid tissue composed of CD3-positive T cells, frequently associated with germinal centers formed by B cells. The differential diagnosis is essentially with serous cystadenoma and mature teratoma. These cysts have no malignant potential.

Mature teratoma is a benign extragonadal germ cell tumor with mature tissues derived from all three germinal layers [31]. They have no gender predominance; the mean age of these patients is 29 years. Macroscopically they present both solid and cystic areas, with frequent calcifications. Microscopically, the cystic spaces are lined by squamous epithelium, admixed with respiratory and columnar epithelium. Suppurative inflammation is frequently present. Mature teratomas have no malignant potential.

References

1. Frantz V (1959) Tumours of the pancreas. Washington, DC: Armed Forces Institute of Pathology
2. Sakorafas GH et al (2011) Primary pancreatic cystic neoplasms of the pancreas revisited. Part IV: Rare cystic neoplasms. Surgical Oncology [Epub ahead of print]
3. Martin RC, Klimstra DS, Brennan MF et al (2002) Solidpseudopapillary tumor of the pancreas: a surgical enigma? Ann Surg Oncol 9:35-40
4. Capellari JO, Geisinger KR, Albertson DA et al (1990) Malignant papillary cystic tumor of the pancreas. Cancer 66:193-198
5. Matsunou H, Konishi F (1990) Papillary-cystic neoplasm of the pancreas: a clinicopathologic study concerning the tumor aging and malignancy of nine cases. Cancer 65:283-291
6. Sclafani LM, Reuter VE, Coit DG, Brennan MF (1991) The malignant nature of papillary and cystic neoplasm of the pancreas. Cancer 68:153-158
7. Nishihara K, Nagoshi M, Tsuneyoshi M et al (1993) Papillary cystic tumors of the pancreas. Assessment of their malignant potential. Cancer 71:82-92
8. Klimstra DS, Wenig BM, Heffess CS (2000) Solid-pseudopapillary tumor of the pancreas: A typically cystic carcinoma of low malignant potential. Semin Diagn Pathol 17:66-80
9. Compagno J, Oertel JE, Kremzar M (1979) Solid and papillary epithelial neoplasm of the pancreas, probably of small duct origin: a clinicopathologic study of 52 cases. Lab Invest 40:248-249.
10. Matsunou H, Konishi F (1990) Papillary-cystic neoplasm of the pancreas: a clinicopathologic study concerning the tumor aging and malignancy of nine cases. Cancer 65:283-291
11. Lam KY, Lo CY, Fan ST (1999) Pancreatic solid-cystic-papillary tumor: clinicopathologic features in eight patients from Hong Kong and review of the literature.World J Surg 23:1045-1050
12. Ferrari L, Seregni E, Bajetta E et al (1999) The biological characteristics of chromogranin A and its role as a circulating marker in neuroendocrine tumours. Anticancer Res 19:3415-3427
13. Falconi MB, Bassi C, Salvia R, Pederzoli P (2003) Clinical manifestation and therapeutic management of non functioning endocrine tumours. In: Procacci CM, Megibow AJ (eds). Imaging of the Pancreas. Cystic and Rare Tumors. Springer pp 153-160
14. Ng KH, Tan PH, Thng CH et al (2003) Solid pseudopapillary tumour of the pancreas. ANZ J Surg 73:410-415
15. Ros PR, Mortele KJ (2001) Imaging features of pancreatic neoplasms. Jbr-Btr 84:239-249
16. Cavallini A, Butturini G, Daskalaki D et al (2011) Laparoscopic Pancreatectomy for Solid Pseudo-Papillary Tumors of the Pancreas is a Suitable Technique; Our Experience with Long-Term Follow-up and Review of the Literature. Ann Surg Oncol 18:352-357
17. Kim CW, Han DJ, Kim J et al (2011) Solid pseudopapillary tumor of the pancreas: Can malignancy be predicted? Surgery 149:625-634
18. Goh BK, Tan YM, Cheow PC et al (2007) Solid pseudopapillary neoplasms of the pancreas: an updated experience. J Surg Oncol 95:640e4
19. Papavramidis T, Papavramidis S (2005) Solid pseudopapillary tumors of the pancreas: review of 718 patients reported in English literature. J Am Coll Surg 200:965e72
20. Zamboni G, Terris B, Scarpa A et al (2002) Acinar cell cystadenoma of the pancreas: a new entity? Am J Surg Pathol 26:698-704

4 Solid-pseudopapillary, Acinar, and Other Cystic Neoplasms

21. Cantrell BB, Cubilla AL, Erlandson RA et al (1981) Acinar cell cystadenocarcinoma of human pancreas. Cancer 47:410-416
22. Ishizaki A, Koito K, Namieno T et al (1995) Acinar cell carcinoma of the pancreas: a rare case of an alpha-fetoprotein-producing cystic tumor. Eur J Radiol 21:58-60
23. Joubert M, Fiche M, Hamy A et al (1998) Extension of an acinar cell pancreatic carcinoma with cystic changes invading the Wirsung canal [in French]. Gastroenterol Clin Biol 22:465-468
24. Stamm B, Burger H, Hollinger A (1987) Acinar cell cystadenocarcinoma of the pancreas. Cancer 60:2542-2547
25. Cantrell BB, Cubilla AL, Erlandson RA et al (1981) Acinar cell cystadenocarcinoma of human pancreas. Cancer 47:410-416
26. Klimstra DS (2007) Nonductal neoplasms of the pancreas. Mod Pathol 20:S94-S112
27. Pogany AC, Kerlan RK Jr, Karam JH et al (1984) Cystic insulinoma. AJR Am J Roentgenol 142:951-952
28. Adsay NV, Klimstra DS (2000) Cystic forms of typically solid pancreatic tumors. Semin Diagn Pathol 17:81-88
29. Iacono C, Serio G, Fugazzola C et al (1992) Cystic islet cell tumors of the pancreas. A clinico-pathological report of two nonfunctioning cases and review of the literature. Int J Pancreatol 11:199-208
30. Iacono C, Cracco N, Zamboni G et al (1996) Lymphoepithelial cyst of the pancreas. Report of two cases and review of the literature. Int J Pancreatol 19:71-76
31. Iacono C, Zamboni G, Di Marcello R et al (1993) Dermoid cyst of the head of the pancreas area. Int J Pancreatol 14:269-273

Intraductal Papillary Mucinous Neoplasms

5

Isabella Frigerio, Giuseppe Zamboni, Riccardo Manfredi, Antonio Pea, Silvia Pennacchio, Eugene Lim and Roberto Salvia

5.1 Introduction

After 30 years during which intraductal papillary mucinous neoplasms (IPMNs) were considered to be rare neoplasms of the pancreas, we now know that they represent a specific entity that is seen in daily clinical practice. This awareness has highlighted the need for an improved understanding of pancreatic diseases. In fact, nowadays, IPMNs are the most frequent cystic neoplasm of the pancreas; this is the case ev en in asymptomatic patients, in whom they are detected as an incidental finding [1]. In our experience, IPMNs are one of the most common indications for pancreatic resection.

Since the first report by Ohashi, in 1982 [2], knowledge of this emerging disease has significantly improved, to the extent that it has been included in the classification of exocrine pancreatic neoplasms proposed by the World Health Organization (WHO), beginning in 1996 [3]. The WHO defines IPMNs as intraductal papillary mucinous neoplasms with tall, columnar, mucin-containing epithelium, with or without papillary projections, involving the main pancreatic duct and/or its branch ducts. In the two decades since this description, updates of the WHO classification have been published, first in 2000 [4] and again in 2010 [5]. Consequently, some authors now distinguish two different entities among intraductal neoplasms according to the site of origin: main duct-IPMN (MD-IPMN) and the less-aggressive branch duct-IPMN (BD-IPMN) [6, 7].

The first guidelines on the management of mucinous tumors of the pancreas were developed during a consensus conference held in Sendai, Japan, in 2005.

I. Frigerio (✉)
Surgery Unit, Casa di cura "Dr. P. Pederzoli",
Peschiera del Garda (VR), Italy
e-mail: isifrigerio@yahoo.com

P. Pederzoli and C. Bassi (eds.), *Uncommon Pancreatic Neoplasms*,
Updates in Surgery
DOI: 10.1007/978-88-470-2673-5_5, © Springer-Verlag Italia 2013

5.2 Epidemiology

The diagnosis of IPMN has significantly improved in the last 15 years but the true incidence of these neoplasms is unknown. It is clear that IPMNs occurred before 1982, but they were misclassified as mucinous cystic neoplasms or mucinous ductal cancers and probably also misdiagnosed as chronic pancreatitis. The increased incidental diagnosis of these cystic lesions, their unification under the common name of IPMN, and the acceptance by clinicians of this new terminology has enabled an estimation of its incidence in patients undergoing resection, for whom the reported value is around 0.8/10 [8]. A slightly higher incidence in men is widely accepted, while patients undergoing resection are typically in the 6th decade of life, in both men and women [9].

Recently some authors have reported a higher incidence of extrapancreatic neoplasms among patients with IPMNs than in either patients with other pancreatic disorders or in the general population [10, 11]. If we consider patients with pancreatic adenocarcinoma (PADC) and those with IPMN, the risk for colonic adenomatous polyps, Barret's metaplasia, and urinary tract malignancies is significantly higher in the IPMN group. There is no difference regarding malignant tumors that have a high incidence in the general population (skin, breast, colorectal, and lung cancers). A group from the Mayo Clinic was the first to show a higher incidence of malignant and benign neoplasms, the latter being possible precursors of future malignancies. To explain this higher incidence, two hypotheses have been formulated: the increased medical surveillance of patients with IPMN (often incidentally diagnosed), and common genetic or extragenomic risk factors for both IPMN and extrapancreatic neoplasms. Another interesting finding is that the majority of extrapancreatic neoplasms are detected before or coincidently with IPMN. However, before a screening program aimed at the early detection of colonic, esophageal, or urinary malignant diseases in IPMN patients can be established, further data are needed.

5.3 Pathology

As noted above, the new 2010 WHO classification recognizes two different entities: MD-IPMN and BD-IPMN. The former are characterized by involvement of the main pancreatic duct, with or without associated involvement of the branch ducts (combined or mixed IPMNs). MD-IPMN usually presents as a dilated ($\geq$ 1 cm) main pancreatic duct filled with mucus that may extrude through a bulging ampulla. In some cases, this appearance may mimic that of a cyst along the main pancreatic duct. MD-IPMNs are usually located in the proximal portion of the gland (75%) but they can spread to the rest of the main pancreatic duct; BD-IPMNs more commonly involve the uncinate process, even if they have been described in the whole gland, as well as in the head, neck, and distal pancreas. In BD-IPMNs, the side branches of the pancreatic ductal system are involved. These neoplasms appear as a cystic lesion communicating with a non-dilated main pancreatic duct. The communication might be macroscopically demonstrable or not; this is usually related to the amount of mucus produced.

Multifocal involvement of the gland by two or more BD-IPMNs is not an uncommon finding. In recent years the diagnosis of multifocal IPMNs at our institution has dramatically increased, whereas metachronous IPMN may reflect either multifocality or a "field defect," predisposing the entire ductal epithelium to the development of this neoplasm.

Non-invasive IPMNs are classified into three categories based on the highest degree of cytoarchitectural atypia: low-grade dysplasia, moderate dysplasia, and high-grade dysplasia/carcinoma in-situ. Invasive neoplasms are classified as IPMN with associated invasive carcinoma. At least four cell-types have been described, according to their histology and mucin immunophenotype:
1. MUC2+, CDX2+: intestinal type (Fig. 5.1 a, b)
2. MUC2-/CDX2-/MUC1+: pancreatobiliary (Fig. 5.2 a, b)

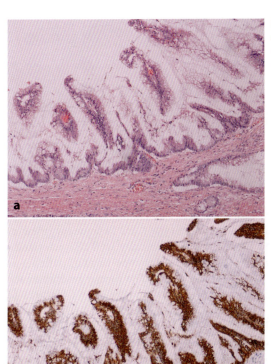

Fig. 5.1 Intraductal papillary mucinous neoplasm (IPMN), intestinal type papillae, with moderate dysplasia (**a**) and MUC2-positivity (**b**)

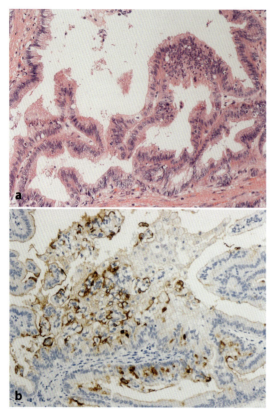

Fig. 5.2 IPMN, pancreatobiliary type papillae, with severe dysplasia (a) and MUC1-positivity (b)

3 MUC5AC+/ MUC6+ and MUC1-/MUC2-/CDX2-: gastric foveolar type (Fig. 5.3a, b)
4 MUC1+/MUC2+/CDX2-: oncocytic types (Fig. 5.4)

Patients with the first type have a good prognosis while those with the second type have a poorer prognosis. In the third type there is frequent involvement of branch ducts; the fourth type is not yet clinically well characterized.

The invasive component, present in approximately one-third of patients, is either a tubular or a mucinous invasive component. The former resembles the conventional ductal carcinoma (Fig. 5.5), while the latter shows features of colloid (mucinous non-cystic) carcinoma (Fig. 5.6). Although MUC2+ intestinal IPMNs can be considered as precursors of MUC2+ mucinous non-cystic carcinoma, characterized by good prognosis, MUC2-/MUC1+ pancreatobiliary IPMNs appear to be closely associated with an aggressive tubular carcinoma [12, 13]. The progression from benign IPMN to malignancy can be radiologically detected, considering either the increase in the diameter of the main duct or the cyst, or the emergence of a mural nodule [14].

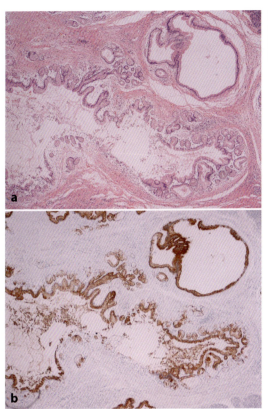

Fig. 5.3 IPMN-branch-duct, gastric type, of the uncinate process, with low-grade dysplasia (**a**) and MUC5AC-positivity (**b**)

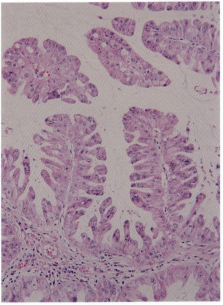

Fig. 5.4 IPMN-oncocytic type. The papillary proliferations are lined by cells with a finely granular cytoplasm and containing nuclei with prominent nucleoli

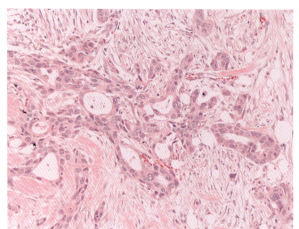

Fig. 5.5 IPMN with tubular-type carcinoma, characterized by infiltrating, irregular tubular structures, similar to those of ordinary ductal carcinoma

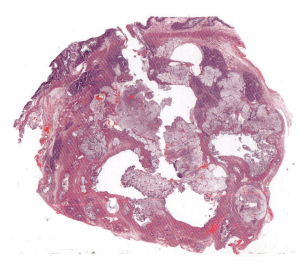

Fig. 5.6 IPMN with "muconodular" carcinomatous transformation. Whole-mount macrosection from a duodenopancreatectomy shows multiple areas of nodular gelatinous carcinomatous tissue

Interestingly, IPMNs can be associated with familial syndromes. For example, they have been detected in asymptomatic family members of patients with familial pancreatic cancer [15], in patients with Peutz-Jeghers syndrome (PJS), with inactivation of the *STK11/LKB1* gene [16], and in association with familial adenomatous polyposis (FAP) [17]. These findings highlight that in patients with IPMN screening for curable pancreatic neoplasia may be possible.

In our experience in collaboration with the Massachusetts General Hospital, among 140 patients with MD-IPMNs who were treated by resection, 12% had adenoma, 28% borderline disease, 12% carcinoma in situ, and 42% invasive carcinoma. Similar data have been reported by other authors [18, 19].

Tanaka et al. found that MD- and BD-IPMNs were associated with malignancy in 70% and 25% of the cases, respectively, while the rate of invasive carcinoma was 43% for MD-IPMN and 15% for the BD type. Thus, these two neoplasms seem to have a significantly different biological behavior, which may influence clinical decision-making with regard to the appropriate management of these two entities.

Moreover, it is not uncommon to recognize different degrees of dysplasia within the same surgical specimen. In our experience, the average age of patients with malignant MD-IPMN is 6.4 years older than that of patients with adenoma or borderline tumor; these observations support the theory of a clonal progression to malignancy in this variant [20].

5.4 Genetics

Regarding the molecular pathogenesis of IPMNs, *KRAS* activating mutations have been identified as an early event that increases in occurrence according to the histological severity of the neoplasm. Mutations in the *KRAS*, *p16*, and *p53* genes are present but are less common in IPMN than in ductal carcinoma, and *DPC4* loss is usually not detected. In a study of 23 cases of resected IPMNs, Wada et al. showed that 65% had a *KRAS* mutation. A loss of heterozygosity (LOH) in 9p21 (p16) increased from 12.5% in adenomas to 75% for carcinomas while LOH in 17p13 (p53) was present only in invasive carcinomas [20]. These results suggest LOH in 9p21 (p16) as an "early" event and LOH in 17p13 (p53) as a later event, providing additional support for a clonal progression process.

A recent report showed that DNA damage checkpoint activation due to *CHK2* inactivation occurs in the early stage of IPMN and seems to prevent its progression whereas p53 accumulation was mostly detected in malignant IPMNs. It was suggested that the DNA damage checkpoint exerts selective pressure on the p53 mutation and that a disturbance of CHK2 inactivation or p53 mutation contributes to the carcinogenesis of IPMNs.

Several other genetic alterations have also been reported in IPMNs. *AKT/PKB* and *HER2/EGFR* activation has been demonstrated in a large portion of these neoplasms, while *CDKN2A/P16* expression is frequently lost, suggesting a correlation with the hypermethylation of the promoter region of P16, more frequently detected in high-grade neoplasms. Some IPMNs show abrogation of *TP53*, especially those with high-grade atypia [21-26]. Despite frequent hemizygous or homozygous deletions of chromosome 18q, *SMAD4* is completely retained in IPMNs [27, 28].

Mutation of *STK11/LKB1*, a PJS gene, and the abrogated expression of *DUSP6/MKP-3*, a gene identified in the deleted region 12q21-q22, suggest a role for these molecules in the development of a subset of IPMNs [29, 30]. Aberrant hypermethylation of at least one CpG island is detected in about 80% of IPMNs, with the overall number of methylated loci significantly higher in high-grade tumors. Genes encoding cyclin D2, TFPI-2 and SOCS-1 have been reported as aberrantly methylated in IPMNs [31].

Global gene expression analysis performed for IPMNs revealed that many of the overexpressed genes are also highly expressed in pancreatic ductal adenocarcinomas. In addition, gene expression profiles evidenced the up-regulation of the genes encoding members of the trefoil factor family (TFF1 and TFF3), CLD4, CXCR4, S100A4, and mesothelin. Some of the encoded proteins have been suggested to play a role in the progression to the invasive form of IPMNs [32-34]; among the underexpressed genes in IPMNs, *CDKN1C/P57KIP2* has been shown to be epigenetically down-regulated.

Recent investigations suggest the involvement of the sonic hedgehog (SHH) pathway in the tumorigenesis of IPMN and that SHH measurement of pancreatic juice may provide some advantages in the treatment or follow-up of a subset of patients with these tumors. The study by Ohuchida et al. [35] provides an outstanding survey of the SHH pathway involvement of IPMN, with its possible clinical implications. The involvement of this pathway was further supported by the report of Jang et al. [36] in their study of the immunohistochemical expression of SHH in IPMNs.

Fascin expression was found to be significantly higher in borderline neoplasms and carcinomas than in adenomas, suggesting that overexpression is involved in the progression of IPMNs. Thus, fascin could become a new therapeutic target for the inhibition of IPMN progression or, at least in the short term, a prognostic marker of IPMN [37].

PIK3CA mutations have been reported in 11% of IPMNs, providing evidence that the oncogenic properties of this gene contribute to these neoplasms [38].

Recent results suggest that HTERT expression in epithelial cells is an indicator of malignant transformation in IPMN. Immunohistochemical detection of HTERT in cells derived from pancreatic juice may therefore ´provide a powerful diagnostic tool and, in this case, a marker of the malignant progression of IPMN [39].

MUC4 and MUC5AC were recently evaluated as potential markers in distinguishing more aggressive IPMNs from less malignant ones, in a study by Kanno et al. [40].

5.5 Clinical Presentation

There are no signs or symptoms suggestive of IPMNs. Patients with MD-IPMN are more often symptomatic, complaining of abdominal pain, pancreatitis, steatorrhea, jaundice, diabetes, or weight loss [41]. Even though some patients with BD-IPMN may present with the above-described symptoms, most are asymptomatic and the neoplasms are incidentally detected during a radiological work-up performed for unrelated problems [42, 43].

It is remarkable that, unlike in pancreatic adenocarcinoma, jaundice is an uncommon presentation of IPMN and occurs only in 15–20% of patients. Jaundice and steatorrhea at presentation are a cause for concern as together they are associated with a much higher incidence of malignant IPMN (8- and 5- fold, respectively). A recent onset or worsening of diabetes is more common in patients with IPMNs with invasive carcinoma (3-fold). In our experience, patients with benign IPMNs had a higher frequency of abdominal pain and a longer duration of symptoms.

5.6 Diagnostic Work-up

Previously, Ohhashi's triad, consisting of a bulging ampulla of Vater, mucin secretion, and dilated main pancreatic duct, was an indicator of IPMN. Today, the great majority of IPMNs are characterized on cross-sectional imaging study, such as computed tomography (CT) or magnetic resonance cholangiopancreatography (MRCP). The radiological and endoscopic features of IPMNs vary according to the morphologic type of the neoplasm. The typical feature of MD-IPMNs is dilatation of the main pancreatic duct > 1cm (Fig. 5.7), eventually extending into the secondary branches, which may appear as cysts (Fig. 5.8). The dilatation can involve the duct of the distal pancreas or, if it is located in the head or in the uncinate process, may be present throughout because of an obstructive effect. BD-IPMN appears as cysts or a cluster of cysts without dilatation of the main duct and is more commonly located in the head-uncinate process. Between 39% and 64% of BD-IPMNs are multifocal (Fig. 5.9a, b).

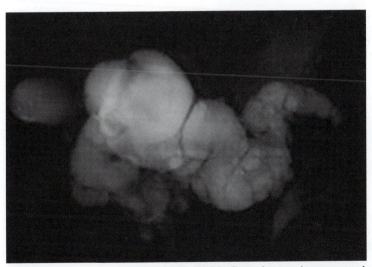

Fig. 5.7 Main pancreatic duct IPMN (MD-IPMN). Coronal magnetic resonance cholangio-pancreatography (MRCP) shows diffuse dilatation of the main pancreatic duct due to the involvement of the entire pancreatic ductal system

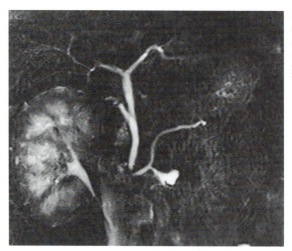

Fig. 5.8 Side-branch IPMN (SB-IPMN). Coronal MRCP shows a cystic dilatation of a side branch in the head of the pancreas, connected with the Wirsung duct

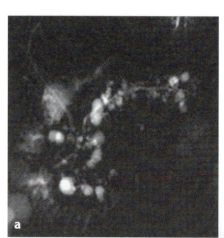

Fig. 5.9 Multifocal SB-IPMN. Coronal MRCP shows a cystic dilatation of multiple side branches located along the whole pancreas (**a**). Axial T2-weighted image shows the connection between the cystically dilated side branches and the main pancreatic duct (**b**)

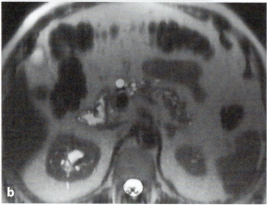

5 Intraductal Papillary Mucinous Neoplasms

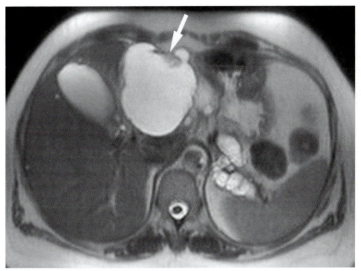

Fig. 5.10 MD-IPMN: mural nodule. Axial T2-weighted image shows dilatation of the main pancreatic duct, with a mural nodule on the non-dependent wall of the duct (*arrow*), indicative of malignant IPMN, which was surgically confirmed

Calcifications are detected in 11% of cases. Nodules and papillary projections, which are significantly associated with the presence of a malignant neoplasm, usually appear as filling defects within the cystic lesions (Fig. 5.10). The pancreatic gland may be enlarged, with signs of pancreatitis, or it may be atrophic. CT and MRCP can localize the tumor and assess its relationship with nearby vessels and other organs. MRCP is particularly useful in the characterization of single or multifocal BD-IPMNs, given the ability of this imaging technique to demonstrate a communication between the main duct and the cyst.

At our institution, in the initial assessment of patients with suspected IPMN we additionally use contrast-enhanced ultrasound (US), which is able to identify and characterize the "cysts" in detail [44].

In those cases in which the diagnosis is uncertain, endoscopic ultrasound (EUS) may be helpful, as it can well identify the dilated main pancreatic duct. In addition, EUS demonstrates the morphological details of any solid component, nodules, or small projections, in the main duct and/or in the cyst communicating with it. EUS is also a safe method for fluid sampling and targeted biopsies by fine-needle aspiration or core biopsy. Examination of fluid sampled from an IPMN provides diagnostic information about the tumor, revealing its viscous aspect, the presence of mucin or mucinous cells, and carcinoembryonic antigen levels [45]. However, it is important to keep in mind that the puncture is done through the gastric or duodenal wall, potentially allowing the needle to carry tumor cells.

Cytologic examination of the pancreatic juice and the subsequent detection of a *KRAS* mutation can also be helpful and, to a limited extent, may predict the likelihood of malignancy, even though this procedure has a low sensitivity (< 20%). More recent work has shown that high-grade atypia on cytology has a sensitivity of 72% for malignancy for all mucinous cysts (mostly IPMN) [46]. We consider EUS as a second-level procedure that should be performed only in selected cases.

In recent years, intraductal endoscopy and/or peroral pancreatoscopy have been introduced but experience is limited and further studies are needed.

Blood tests that include tumor markers are mandatory, with measurements of CEA, Ca19-9, and Ca125.

Clinical history, radiology, and endoscopy should contribute to obtaining a correct diagnosis of IPMN and to differentiate it from other cystic neoplasms, such as serous cystadenoma or mucinous cystic neoplasms, and from other cystic lesions of the pancreas (pseudocyst, true pancreatic cyst). Once IPMN is identified, the following step is the differential diagnosis between MD- and BD-IPMN and the determination of those parameters associated with a high risk of malignancy. Jaundice, steatorrhea and new or worsening diabetes should raise suspicion for degeneration. A lesion > 30 mm in diameter, a dilated main pancreatic duct (> 10 mm), and the presence of nodules, thick walls, or papillary projections are morphological aspects that should always alert clinicians [47].

5.7 Management

During the consensus conference held in Sendai in 2005, a group of surgeons, gastroenterologists and pathologists edited the first guidelines pertaining to the management of IPMNs. Before 2005, all patients with a diagnosis of IPMN were considered to be at risk of developing malignancy, and therefore surgery was always proposed. Since the Sendai meeting, two different approaches have been defined when considering MD-IPMN (including the mixed form) and BD-IPMN.

5.7.1 Main Duct-IPMNs

Patients with MD-IPMN or the mixed form, when surgically fit, should always be candidates for resection because of the high prevalence of in situ and invasive carcinoma found in resected specimens (70%). Of note is the observation that in patients with MD-IPMNs there may be malignancy regardless of the presence or absence of symptoms. Accordingly, the radiological aspect of these lesions can determine the indication for surgery.

The surgical management of MD-IPMNs is challenging. While in other pancreatic tumors preoperative imaging can accurately locate the tumor and

5 Intraductal Papillary Mucinous Neoplasms

thereby allow the planning of a pancreatic resection, this is not always the case in MD-IPMNs. Segmental dilatation of the main duct, as seen on preoperative studies, may occur both proximal and distal to the tumor, because of mucus overproduction. In such case, localization of the neoplasm is more difficult.

A typical resection (pancreaticoduodenectomy, left pancreatectomy, total pancreatectomy, according to the site and extension of the disease) with lymph node dissection is mandatory. Limited resections, such as middle pancreatectomy, have been proposed for MD-IPMN, but in our experience with MD-IPMN patients this results in a high rate of positive resection margins and recurrences, with similar results reported by other authors [48]. Consequently, in this setting we recommend standard resections. Since IPMN extends along the pancreatic duct and may do so without macroscopic tumor, it is important to exclude residual tumor on frozen section [49].

Three different aspects of the ductal mucosa can be detected by analyzing the surgical margin: (1) normal ductal epithelium in the main duct means that radical resection has been achieved; (2) de-epithelialized or a denuded epithelium should not be considered as a negative margin since local recurrence is also possible; (3) adenoma, borderline, or carcinoma requires an extension of the surgical resection up to total pancreatectomy.

In cases of de-epithelialization, adenoma, or borderline tumor at the surgical margin, the optimal surgical strategy is controversial: we usually extend the resection by a few centimeters to obtain a new margin, aiming to achieve a negative resection margin. In our experience involving 140 patients with MD-IPMN who underwent surgical resection, the rate of negative margins in the surgical specimen was 58.5%, and the results of the intraoperative frozen section analysis modified the surgical plan, leading to an extension of the resection or to total pancreatectomy in 29 patients (20.7%) [50].

Recurrence in the pancreatic remnant may develop even if the transection margin is negative and even in patients with noninvasive disease. The presence of a positive resection margin, multicentric IPMNs with synchronous skip lesions along the main duct that are still present (but not detectable) at the time of surgery, and metachronous lesions (given that IPMN may be a marker of a "field defect" associated with a propensity for tumor development) may explain recurrence in the pancreatic remnant after the resection of a MD-IPMN.

For all these reasons, the role of total pancreatectomy in IPMN must be carefully evaluated and tailored to each single patient. Some authors have reported that for malignant IPMNs the frequency of recurrence (local recurrence or distant metastases) is similar whether or not total pancreatectomy is performed [51, 52]; Chari et al. reported a recurrence rate of 62% after total pancreatectomy and of 67% after partial pancreatectomy [19]. The risks and long-term complications of total pancreatectomy must be considered and discussed with patients. Finally, in patients with MD-IPMN undergoing pylorus-preserving pancreaticoduodenectomy, pancreaticogastrostomy may be preferred instead of pancreaticojejunostomy because it allows direct endoscopic access to the pancreatic stump during follow-up, leaving open the possibility of pancreatic juice sampling for cytological examination [53].

5.7.2 Branch-Duct IPMNs

The prevalence of malignancy is much lower (25%) in BD-IPMNs than in MD-IPMNs and it is predictable on the basis of symptoms, tumor size, and morphological criteria. Thus, a strict follow-up is advocated for patients with BD-IPMN < 3 cm, with no nodules or duct dilatation (which would imply a combined IPMN). Follow-up consists of MRCP repeated 6 months after the first diagnosis and then yearly, together with measurement of Ca19-9 levels, unless there is an increase in size, the development of nodules, or the onset of symptoms. It should be emphasized that this non-operative approach should be carried out in experienced centers and that data from large series are still needed for its validation (Fig. 5.11a, b).

In our earlier experience of 109 patients with BD-IPMN [54], 20 patients (18.3%) underwent immediate surgery because of the presence of symptoms

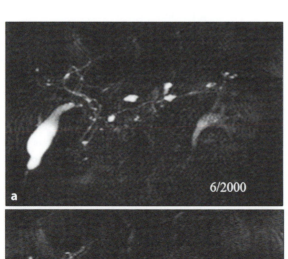

Fig. 5.11 SB-IPMN evolution. Coronal MRCP obtained in June 2000 shows multifocal side-branch IPMNs. The number and size of the dilated side branches were unchanged in May 2005

5 Intraductal Papillary Mucinous Neoplasms

and/or parameters associated with malignancy. A pathological diagnosis of BD-IPMN was always confirmed; an invasive carcinoma was diagnosed in two patients (10%) and a carcinoma in situ in one (5%). Eighty-nine patients (81.7%) were followed for a median of 32 months. After a mean follow-up of 18.2 months, in five patients (5.6%) an increase in size of the lesion was determined and surgery was performed. The pathological diagnosis was branch-duct adenoma in three patients and borderline in two. None of the patients had malignant changes on follow-up. This study suggests that in very selected cases a non-operative approach is safe and feasible. It also provides further evidence that the biological behavior of BD-IPMN is different than that of the main-duct type.

Other authors have described similar experiences in the conservative management of BD-IPMN. Cauley et al. [55] followed 244 patients with BD-IPMN (described as low risk IPMN); in this group, 32 patients (12%) developed a new indication for resection and two (1%) developed invasive cancer during a mean surveillance of 35 months. No patient with an increasing size of the cyst developed malignancy. In a follow-up of 103 patients, Sawai et al. [56] reported that progression to invasive cancer occurred in 3.9%.

With more data emerging in the literature, it appears that cyst size does not correlate well with the risk of malignancy [57, 58]. The threshold of 3 cm for observing BD-IPMN is currently under scrutiny. According to Markov-based normograms in guiding the indication for surgery, a cyst size > 2 cm favours overall survival regardless of quality of life (QOL), but with a QOL-adjusted survival a 3-cm threshold is more appropriate [59]. This has prompted calls for a review of the Sendai criteria for observing BD-IPMNs. The Heidelberg unit has suggested that only BD-IPMN cysts < 1–1.5 cm should be observed for surgically fit patients [60]. Clearly, controversies remain regarding the best treatment strategies for patients with BD-IPMNs [61]

In terms of the surgical approach, a typical resection should be performed for BD-IPMNs. For asymptomatic patients with a small single lesion (< 3 cm) at the neck of the pancreas, without any suspicion for malignancy, a middle pancreatectomy is an option. In the case of multifocal disease, a total pancreatectomy or an extended standard resection ensures radical treatment; however, a more selective approach can be considered, with segmental resection of the largest lesion (or of the lesion "suspected" of malignancy) and non-operative management with strict follow-up of the remnant BD-IPMN.

Indications for surgery in multifocal BD-IPMN follow the same rules as established for uni-focal BD-IPMN: symptomatic patients and suspicion of malignancy.

5.7.3 Combined IPMNs

The origin of the mixed form of IPMNs is unknown; that is, whether they originate from MD-IPMN or arise as a combined form. Regardless of their pathogenesis, their biological behavior is known to be similar to that of MD-IPMNs and their treatment follows the same rules: high risk of malignant change and, for all surgically fit patients, an indication for surgery [62].

5.8 Post-operative Follow-up

After resection, strict follow-up is necessary. Patients with malignant IPMN have an obviously higher risk of recurrence, but neoplastic recurrence can arise even in the presence of a benign tumor with negative resection margins, particularly for MD-IPMNs. It is important to detect a recurrence or the development of a new disease in the remnant since this is an indication for a second resection. In our experience with 140 patients with MD-IPMN who underwent resection, eight (7%) developed a recurrence in the remnant. Of these, seven had invasive carcinoma at initial histology and one had an adenoma with negative resection margins; this patient underwent a completion pancreatectomy for carcinoma in situ.

In our opinion, clinical examination, biochemical assessment, and US, CT, or MRCP—performed every 6 months in patients with malignant tumors and yearly for those with benign IPMNs—offers a safe follow-up approach. In patients with multifocal BD-IPMN treated by partial pancreatectomy, strict follow-up should be performed to evaluate the remnant gland or lesions in the remaining pancreas and the eventual development of new lesions. MRCP is particularly useful in this setting [63].

5.9 Prognosis

The survival of patients with IPMN, even when malignant and invasive, is always better than that of patients with pancreatic ductal adenocarcinoma. In our experience, based on a follow-up of 137 patients treated by resection, 5- and 10-year disease specific survival (DSS) for 80 patients with adenoma, borderline, and in situ carcinoma was 100%, while for 57 patients with invasive carcinoma the DSS was 60% and 50%, respectively. In another large series, the 5-year DSS for patients with IPMN with invasive carcinoma ranged from 36% to 43% [64].

In a recent study [65] based on a multivariate analysis, we identified three independent factors associated with poor prognosis in invasive IPMN carcinoma: Ca19-9 value > 37 U/ml (adjusted for jaundice), a family history of pancreatic cancer, and a lymph node ratio (LNR) > 0.2. These three factors are associated with a 5-year survivals of 44.2%, 16.7%, and 11%, respectively. However, it is still difficult to define the impact on clinical practice of these prognostic factors. Only a family history and Ca19-9 levels can be determined preoperatively and are therefore able to influence decision-making, for example, in those patients with BD-IPMN in whom surgery may not be the first option. Our current strategy is to recommend early surgery for patients with high-risk lesions; the early detection of signs of malignancy or recurrence may be prognostically beneficial for these patients.

References

1. Carbognin G, Zamboni G, Pinali L et al (2006) Branch duct IPMTs: value of cross-sectional imaging in the assessment of biological behavior and follow-up. Abdom Imaging 31:320-325
2. Ohashi K. MY, Murayama M (1982) Four cases of mucus secreting pancreatic cancer. Prog Dig Endoscopy 20:348-351
3. Kloppel G SE, Capella C, Longnecker DS (1996) Histological typing of tumours of the exocrine pancreas. World Health Organization International Histological Classification of Tumours. Springer-Verlag, Berlin
4. Longnecker DS AG, Hruban RH, Kloppel G (2000) Intraductal papillary-mucinous neoplasms of the pancreas in Hamilton SR, Aaltonen LA(eds): World Health Organization classification of tumors. pathology and genetics of tumors of the digestive system. IARC, Lyon, pp. 237-241
5. Adsay NV, Fukushima N, Furukawa T et al (2010) Intraductal neoplasms of the pancreas. In: Bosman FT, Carneiro F, Hruban RH, et al (eds) World Health Organization classification of tumours of the digestive system. 4th edn. IARC, Lyon, pp. 304-13
6. Kobari M, Egawa S, Shibuya K et al (1999) Intraductal papillary mucinous tumors of the pancreas comprise 2 clinical subtypes: differences in clinical characteristics and surgical management. Arch Surg 134:1131-1136
7. Terris B, Ponsot P, Paye F et al (2000) Intraductal papillary mucinous tumors of the pancreas confined to secondary ducts show less aggressive pathologic features as compared with those involving the main pancreatic duct. Am J Surg Pathol 24:1372-1377
8. Fernández-del Castillo C, Adsay NV (2010) Intraductal papillary mucinous neoplasms of the pancreas. Gastroenterology 139:708-13
9. Salvia R, Fernandez-del Castillo C, Bassi C et al (2004) Main-duct intraductal papillary mucinous neoplasms of the pancreas: clinical predictors of malignancy and long-term survival following resection. Ann Surg 239:678-685
10. Reid-Lombardo KM, Mathis KL, Wood CM et al (2010) Frequency of extrapancreatic neoplasms in intraductal papillary mucinous neoplasm of the pancreas: implications for management. Ann Surg 251:64-69
11. Baumgaertner I, Corcos O, Couvelard A et al (2008) Prevalence of extrapancreatic cancers in patients with histologically proven intraductal papillary mucinous neoplasms of the pancreas: a case-control study. Am J Gastroenterol 103:2878-2882
12. Luttges J, Zamboni G, Longnecker D, Kloppel G (2001) The immunohistochemical mucin expression pattern distinguishes different types of intraductal papillary mucinous neoplasms of the pancreas and determines their relationship to mucinous noncystic carcinoma and ductal adenocarcinoma. Am J Surg Pathol 25:942-948
13. Adsay NV, Merati K, Basturk O et al (2004) Pathologically and biologically distinct types of epithelium in intraductal papillary mucinous neoplasms: delineation of an "intestinal" pathway of carcinogenesis in the pancreas. Am J Surg Pathol 28:839-848
14. Yamaguchi T, Baba T, Ishihara T et al (2005) Long-term follow-up of intraductal papillary mucinous neoplasm of the pancreas with ultrasonography. Clin Gastroenterol Hepatol 3:1136-1143
15. Canto MI, Goggins M, Hruban RH et al (2006) Screening for early pancreatic neoplasia in high-risk individuals: a prospective controlled study. Clin Gastroenterol Hepatol 4:766-781 quiz 665

16. Su GH, Hruban RH, Bansal RK et al (1999) Germline and somatic mutations of the STK11/LKB1 Peutz-Jeghers gene in pancreatic and biliary cancers. Am J Pathol 154:1835-1840
17. Maire F, Hammel P, Terris B et al (2002) Intraductal papillary and mucinous pancreatic tumour: a new extracolonic tumour in familial adenomatous polyposis. Gut 51:446-449
18. Sohn TA, Yeo CJ, Cameron JL et al (2004) Intraductal papillary mucinous neoplasms of the pancreas: an updated experience. Ann Surg 239:788-797
19. Chari ST, Yadav D, Smyrk TC et al (2002) Study of recurrence after surgical resection of intraductal papillary mucinous neoplasm of the pancreas. Gastroenterology 123:1500-1507
20. Wada K, Takada T, Yasuda H et al (2004) Does "clonal progression" relate to the development of intraductal papillary mucinous tumors of the pancreas? J Gastrointest Surg 8:289-296
21. Satoh K, Shimosegawa T, Moriizumi S et al (1996) K-ras mutation and p53 protein accumulation in intraductal mucin-hypersecreting neoplasms of the pancreas. Pancreas 12:362-368
22. Kitago M, Ueda M, Aiura K et al (2004) Comparison of K-ras point mutation distributions in intraductal papillary-mucinous tumors and ductal adenocarcinoma of the pancreas. Int J Cancer 110:177-182
23. Sessa F, Solcia E, Capella C et al (1994) Intraductal papillary-mucinous tumours represent a distinct group of pancreatic neoplasms: an investigation of tumour cell differentiation and K-ras, p53 and c-erbB-2 abnormalities in 26 patients. Virchows Arch 425:357-367
24. Semba S, Moriya T, Kimura W, Yamakawa M (2003) Phosphorylated Akt/PKB controls cell growth and apoptosis in intraductal papillary-mucinous tumor and invasive ductal adenocarcinoma of the pancreas. Pancreas 26:250-257
25. House MG, Guo M, Iacobuzio-Donahue C, Herman JG (2003) Molecular progression of promoter methylation in intraductal papillary mucinous neoplasms (IPMN) of the pancreas. Carcinogenesis 24:193-198
26. Furukawa T, Fujisaki R, Yoshida Y et al (2005) Distinct progression pathways involving the dysfunction of DUSP6/MKP-3 in pancreatic intraepithelial neoplasia and intraductal papillary-mucinous neoplasms of the pancreas. Mod Pathol 18:1034-1042
27. Inoue H, Furukawa T, Sunamura M et al (2001) Exclusion of SMAD4 mutation as an early genetic change in human pancreatic ductal tumorigenesis. Genes Chrom Cancer 31:295-299
28. Iacobuzio-Donahue CA, Klimstra DS, Adsay NV et al (2000) Dpc-4 protein is expressed in virtually all human intraductal papillary mucinous neoplasms of the pancreas: comparison with conventional ductal adenocarcinomas. Am J Pathol 157:755-761
29. Sato N, Rosty C, Jansen M et al (2001) STK11/LKB1 Peutz-Jeghers gene inactivation in intraductal papillary-mucinous neoplasms of the pancreas. Am J Pathol 159:2017-2022
30. Xu S, Furukawa T, Kanai N et al (2005) Abrogation of DUSP6 by hypermethylation in human pancreatic cancer. J Hum Genet 50:159-167
31. Sato N, Goggins M (2006) Epigenetic alterations in intraductal papillary mucinous neoplasms of the pancreas. J Hepatobiliary Pancreat Surg 13:280-285
32. Terris B, Blaveri E, Crnogorac-Jurcevic T et al (2002) Characterization of gene expression profiles in intraductal papillary-mucinous tumors of the pancreas. Am J Pathol. 160:1745-1754
33. Sato N, Fukushima N, Maitra A et al (2004) Gene expression profiling identifies genes associated with invasive intraductal papillary mucinous neoplasms of the pancreas. Am J Pathol 164:903-914
34. Sato N, Matsubayashi H, Abe T et al (2005) Epigenetic down-regulation of CDKN1C/p57KIP2 in pancreatic ductal neoplasms identified by gene expression profiling. Clin Cancer Res 11:4681-4688
35. Ohuchida K, Mizumoto K, Fujita H et al (2006) Sonic hedgehog is an early developmental marker of intraductal papillary mucinous neoplasms: clinical implications of mRNA levels in pancreatic juice. J Pathol. 210:42-48

5 Intraductal Papillary Mucinous Neoplasms

36. Jang KT, Lee KT, Lee JG et al (2007) Immunohistochemical expression of Sonic hedgehog in intraductal papillary mucinous tumor of the pancreas. Appl Immunohistochem Mol Morphol 15:294-298
37. Yamaguchi H, Inoue T, Eguchi T et al (2007) Fascin overexpression in intraductal papillary mucinous neoplasms (adenomas, borderline neoplasms, and carcinomas) of the pancreas, correlated with increased histological grade. Mod Pathol 20:552-561
38. Schonleben F, Qiu W, Ciau NT et al (2006) PIK3CA mutations in intraductal papillary mucinous neoplasm/carcinoma of the pancreas. Clin Cancer Res 12:3851-3855
39. Hashimoto Y, Murakami Y, Uemura K et al (2008) Detection of human telomerase reverse transcriptase (hTERT) expression in tissue and pancreatic juice from pancreatic cancer. Surgery 143:113-125
40. Kanno A, Satoh K, Kimura K et al (2006) The expression of MUC4 and MUC5AC is related to the biologic malignancy of intraductal papillary mucinous neoplasms of the pancreas. Pancreas 33:391-396
41. Falconi M, Salvia R, Bassi C et al (2001) Clinicopathological features and treatment of intraductal papillary mucinous tumour of the pancreas. Br J Surg 88:376-381
42. Sugiyama M, Izumisato Y, Abe N et al (2003) Predictive factors for malignancy in intraductal papillary-mucinous tumours of the pancreas. Br J Surg 90:1244-1249
43. Rodriguez JR, Salvia R, Crippa S et al (2007) Branch-duct intraductal papillary mucinous neoplasms: observations in 145 patients who underwent resection. Gastroenterology 133:72-79 quiz 309-310
44. Faccioli N, Crippa S, Bassi C, D'Onofrio M (2009) Contrast-enhanced ultrasonography of the pancreas. Pancreatology 9:560-566
45. Brugge WR, Lewandrowski K, Lee-Lewandrowski E et al (2004) Diagnosis of pancreatic cystic neoplasms: a report of the cooperative pancreatic cyst study. Gastroenterology 126:1330-1336
46. Genevay M, Mino-Kenudson M, Yaeger K et al (2011) Cytology adds value to imaging studies for risk assessment for pancreatic mucinous cysts. Ann Surg 254:977-983
47. Sakorafas GH, Sarr MG, van de Velde CJ, Peros G (2005) Intraductal papillary mucinous neoplasms of the pancreas: a surgical perspective. Surg Oncol 14:155-178
48. Crippa S, Bassi C, Warshaw AL et al (2007) Middle pancreatectomy: indications, short- and long-term operative outcomes. Ann Surg 246:69-76
49. Gigot JF, Deprez P, Sempoux C et al (2001) Surgical management of intraductal papillary mucinous tumors of the pancreas: the role of routine frozen section of the surgical margin, intraoperative endoscopic staged biopsies of the Wirsung duct, and pancreaticogastric anastomosis. Arch Surg 136:1256-1262
50. Couvelard A, Sauvanet A, Kianmanesh R et al (2005) Frozen sectioning of the pancreatic cut surface during resection of intraductal papillary mucinous neoplasms of the pancreas is useful and reliable: a prospective evaluation. Ann Surg 242:774-778
51. Jang JY, Kim SW, Ahn YJ et al (2005) Multicenter analysis of clinicopathologic features of intraductal papillary mucinous tumor of the pancreas: is it possible to predict the malignancy before surgery? Ann Surg Oncol 12:124-132
52. Maire F, Hammel P, Terris B et al (2002) Prognosis of malignant intraductal papillary mucinous tumours of the pancreas after surgical resection. Comparison with pancreatic ductal adenocarcinoma. Gut 51:717-722
53. Bassi C, Butturini G, Salvia R et al (2006) Open pancreaticogastrostomy after pancreaticoduodenectomy: a pilot study. J Gastrointest Surg 10:1072-1080
54. Salvia R, Crippa S, Falconi M et al (2007) Branch-duct intraductal papillary mucinous neoplasms of the pancreas: to operate or not to operate? Gut 56:1086-1090
55. Cauley CE, Waters JA, Dumas RP et al (2012) Outcomes of primary surveillance for intraductal papillary mucinous neoplasm. J Gastrointest Surg 16:258-266
56. Pelaez-Luna, M et al (2007) Do consensus indications for resection in branch duct intraductal papillary mucinous neoplasm predict malignancy? A study of 147 patients. Am J Gastroenterol 102:1759-1764

57. Schmidt CM, White PB, Waters JA et al (2007) Intraductal papillary mucinous neoplasms: predictors of malignant and invasive pathology. Ann Surg 246:644-651
58. Schnelldorfer T, Sarr MG, Nagorney DM et al (2008) Experience with 208 resections for intraductal papillary mucinous neoplasm of the pancreas. Arch Surg 143:639-646
59. Weinberg BM, Spiegel BM, Tomlinson JS, Farrell JJ (2010) Asymptomatic pancreatic cystic neoplasms: maximizing survival and quality of life using Markov-based clinical nomograms. Gastroenterology 138:531-540
60. Fritz S, Buchler M.W, Werner J (2012) Surgical therapy of intraductal papillary mucinous neoplasms of the pancreas. Der Chirurg 83:130-135
61. Tanaka M (2011) Controversies in the management of pancreatic IPMN. Nat Rev Gastroenterol Hepatol 8:56-60
62. Crippa S, Fernandez-Del Castillo C, Salvia R et al (2010) Mucin-producing neoplasms of the pancreas: an analysis of distinguishing clinical and epidemiologic characteristics. Clin Gastroenterol Hepatol 8:213-219
63. Pilleul F, Rochette A, Partensky C et al (2005) Preoperative evaluation of intraductal papillary mucinous tumors performed by pancreatic magnetic resonance imaging and correlated with surgical and histopathologic findings. J Magn Reson Imaging 21:237-244
64. D'Angelica M, Brennan MF, Suriawinata AA et al (2004) Intraductal papillary mucinous neoplasms of the pancreas: an analysis of clinicopathologic features and outcome. Ann Surg 239:400-408
65. Partelli S, Fernandez-Del Castillo C, Bassi C et al (2010) Invasive intraductal papillary mucinous carcinomas of the pancreas: predictors of survival and the role of lymph node ratio. Ann Surg. 251:477-482

The Role of the Oncologist in the Diagnosis and Management of Malignant Cystic Neoplasms

6

Alessandra Auriemma, Davide Melisi and Giampaolo Tortora

6.1 Introduction

Cystic tumors are uncommon pancreatic lesions but, at least according to our experience, they account for 30% of radical pancreatic resections. This high frequency can be explained by several reasons but especially by the increasingly widespread use of modern imaging techniques, such that in the clinical workup of unrelated conditions, suspicious cystic pancreatic lesions are often incidentally revealed. The resulting likelihood of early detection has improved the management of these patients.

Thus far, the efficacy of chemo- or radiotherapy in treating malignant cystic tumors has not been demonstrated, leaving surgery as the only therapeutic option. The responsibility of the surgeon in such cases is two-fold, as he or she will be involved in the diagnosis and then in the treatment (resection) of the lesion.

However, for patients in whom surgery is not or not yet an option, close follow-up is mandated. This applies to patients with a benign or indeterminate lesion and to those with coexisting critical conditions. In these patients, the updated WHO classification is useful to understand the relationship between the biological behavior of the tumor and the prognosis. More recently, oncologists have increasingly contributed to the diagnosis and management of patients with malignant cystic neoplasms, as discussed in the following section.

G. Tortora (✉)
Department of Medical Oncology, "G.B. Rossi" University Hospital,
Verona, Italy
e-mail: gianpaolo.tortora@univr.it

P. Pederzoli and C. Bassi (eds.), *Uncommon Pancreatic Neoplasms*,
Updates in Surgery
DOI: 10.1007/978-88-470-2673-5_6, © Springer-Verlag Italia 2013

6.2 The Role of the Oncologist in the Diagnosis and Management of Malignant Cystic Neoplasms

Cystic neoplasms of the pancreas are relatively rare lesions. Most of them are either benign or low-grade indolent neoplasias, with a prognosis significantly better than the dismal outcome of patients with ductal adenocarcinoma [1].

As extensively described elsewhere in this book, cystic neoplasms have been classified by the WHO into four types: serous cystic neoplasms (SCNs), intraductal papillary mucinous neoplasms (IPMNs), mucinous cystic neoplasms (MCNs), and solid pseudopapillary neoplasms (SPNs). This distinction is very important since the four types differ in their malignant potential, which in turn determines their correct management. The mucinous types, i.e., IPMNs and MCNs, are of particular relevance for medical oncologists because of the well-established malignant potential of these tumors.

6.2.1 Serous Cystic Neoplasms

The malignant degeneration of SCNs of the pancreas is very rare. Moreover, the benign and malignant variants have very similar histological appearances, with the only distinguishing characteristic of malignant lesions being their tendency to invade surrounding structure. Metastases to regional lymph nodes, liver, lung, and bone marrow also have been reported. Nonetheless, the prognosis of these patients is very good, and an aggressive surgical approach, when feasible, is the preferred therapeutic approach [2-5] . As noted above, to date, there have been no studies or reports in which chemotherapeutic strategies have been used in this setting.

6.2.2 Mucinous Cystic Neoplasms

In contrast to SCNs, mucinous cystic and intraductal papillary neoplasms share a high tendency to become malignant. At histological evaluation of these tumors, it is common to find all the different steps of tumor progression. Thus, the pathologist must carefully search for foci of carcinoma in situ or invasive carcinoma, neither of which may be visible grossly. Surgery remains the mainstay of cure for patients with MCNs and IPMNs. The timing of surgery and the most appropriate technique are defined based on a multidisciplinary evaluation, considering the preoperative, radiological, and pathological diagnosis, symptoms, size and growth rate of the lesion, and the age and performance status of the patient. When indicated, resection is usually curative. An appropriate follow-up program is then defined based on the risk of recurrence. In selected cases, surgery can be considered also in metastatic disease, as some studies have reported the long-term survival of these patients. As for SCNs, medical oncologists have a marginal role in the management of MCNs and

IPMNs given that, due to the low incidence of malignant and metastatic cystic neoplasms, there are no or only a few clinical studies addressing the efficacy of radio- or chemotherapeutic strategies or the use of common cytotoxic drugs in their treatment.

Several risk factors for malignancy have been defined for patients with MCNs, including tumor size > 4 cm, associated mural nodules, septa, and eggshell calcifications. Surgery, intended as a "standard" pancreatic resection, is the most important and curative approach. If the histological evaluation finds evidence of an invasive carcinoma, a strict follow-up must be programmed, since the risk of recurrence and metastases is high even if the prognosis of these patients is better than that of patients with classical adenocarcinoma, with 5-year survival rates ranging from 15 to 33% [6, 7]. There are a few cases in which mucinous cystadenocarcinoma was detected during pregnancy or in the post-partum period. As MCNs are diagnosed almost exclusively in women, a role for sex hormones in tumorigenesis can be hypothesized. This relationship is also supported by the ovarian-tumor-like stroma that characterizes MCNs. The clinical management in these cases is more complicated, both from the surgical and the oncological point of view [8-10]. Of note, a case of mucinous cystadenocarcinoma during hormone replacement therapy has been reported [11]. It is therefore crucial that women with cystic masses of the pancreas who need hormonal treatment or who wish to become pregnant are carefully monitored, since either of these conditions can be associated with the evolution and transformation of MCN.

Patients with metastatic MCN have a poor prognosis, and they are usually treated according to the same regimen used in patients with adenocarcinoma. Metastatic MCNs can spread to the peritoneum. In one report, a patient with advanced mucinous cystadenocarcinoma with peritoneal dissemination was treated with gemcitabine, with a marked shrinkage of the tumor [12]. In another, intraperitoneal chemotherapy with cisplatin was administered in the treatment of pseudomyxoma peritonei associated with a pancreatic mucinous cystadenocarcinoma, with very good long-term results [13]. A single case of Sister Mary Joseph's nodule, as an umbilical metastasis of mucinous cystadenocarcinoma, was described [14]. In two cases of unresectable cystadenocarcinoma, a combination regimen in which 5-fluorouracil was administered with radiation therapy showed good activity, with marked reduction in tumor size and carcinoembryonic antigen (CEA) levels, allowing subsequent resection of the lesions [15]. Rare tumors, such as anaplastic carcinoma, osteoclast-like giant cell tumor, carcinosarcoma, and undifferentiated carcinoma, can be associated with MCNs; these entities need to be recognized because of their highly aggressive behaviors [16, 17].

A molecular genetic distinction among the various types of cystic neoplasms was recently described, by determining the exon sequences of DNA from the neoplastic epithelium of these tumors. The analysis of only five genes (*VHL, RNF43, CTNNB1, GNAS,* and *KRAS*) was sufficient to distinguish among the different cystic neoplasms [18]. Of note, all five genes encode either components of the E3 ubiquitin ligase complex or proteins that hence become resistant to degradation by this complex. In a separate study, *GNAS* mutations at codon 201 were detected in 66% of the DNA samples isolated from IPMN cyst fluids. Over 96% of these IPMNs had either a *GNAS* or a *KRAS* mutation and more than half had both mutations. Interestingly, most of the invasive adenocarcinomas that developed in association with IPMNs contained *GNAS* mutations. These mutations were not found either in other types of pancreatic cystic neoplasms or in invasive adenocarcinomas not associated with IPMNs, indicating that GNAS mutation provides a novel molecular pathway leading to IPMN-related pancreatic carcinoma [19]. Thus, when combined with clinical and radiological data, molecular genetic profiles could lead to a more accurate diagnosis and to a more patient-tailored treatment plan.

6.2.3 Intraductal Papillary Mucinous Neoplasms

These tumors can be precursors of invasive carcinomas. Their malignant potential differs depending on the origin of the lesion, as those from the main duct (MD-IPMN) have a higher risk of malignancy than those from branch ducts (BD-IPMN). Surgery is crucial in the management of MD-IPMNs but should also be considered in BD-IPMNs > 3 cm in diameter and in IPMNs with nodules or duct dilatation (mixed IPMN), since in this case the malignant potential is higher. There are no data regarding the efficacy of adjuvant therapy in any of the IPMN types [20]. Interestingly, some authors reported a higher incidence of extrapancreatic malignancies and preneoplastic lesions, especially but not exclusively in the gastrointestinal tract, in patients with IPMNs than in the general population. Thus, the oncologist must bear this information in mind with respect to the long-term follow-up of these patients [21].

6.3 Conclusions

There are very few data supporting the use of chemotherapy in the management of patients with pancreatic cystic neoplasms. Adjuvant treatment is not routinely suggested, considering the low incidence of malignancy of these lesions. In the metastatic setting, there are no specific treatments with demonstrated efficacy; therefore, the common chemotherapeutic regimens used for advanced pancreatic adenocarcinoma should be considered in appropriate cases. Nonetheless, surgery is the only therapeutic strategy that can offer high curative rate to patients with malignant pancreatic cystic neoplasms. Accordingly, every patient should be evaluated carefully to determine eligibility for pancreatic resection, based on a multidisciplinary assessment.

References

1. Adsay NV (2008) Cystic neoplasia of the pancreas: pathology and biology. J Gastrointest Surg 12:401-404
2. Cho W, Cho YB, Jang KT et al (2011) Pancreatic serous cystadenocarcinoma with invasive growth into the colon and spleen. J Korean Surg Soc 81:221-224
3. Eriguchi N, Aoyagi S, Nakayama T et al (1998) Serous cystadenocarcinoma of the pancreas with liver metastases. J Hepatobiliary Pancreat Surg 5:467-470
4. King JC, Ng TT, White SC et al (2009) Pancreatic serous cystadenocarcinoma: a case report and review of the literature. J Gastrointest Surg 13:1864-1868
5. Matsumoto, T, Hirano S, Yada K et al (2005) Malignant serous cystic neoplasm of the pancreas: report of a case and review of the literature. J Clin Gastroenterol 39:253-256
6. Grutzmann, R, Niedergethmann M, Pilarsky C et al (2010) Intraductal papillary mucinous tumors of the pancreas: biology, diagnosis, and treatment. Oncologist 15:1294-1309
7. Benarroch-Gampel J, Riall TS (2010) Extrapancreatic malignancies and intraductal papillary mucinous neoplasms of the pancreas. World J Gastrointest Surg 2:363-367
8. Sakorafas GH, Sarr MG (2005) Cystic neoplasms of the pancreas; what a clinician should know. Cancer Treat Rev 31:507-535
9. Sakorafas GH, Smyrniotis V, Reid-Lombardo KM, Sarr MG (2011) Primary pancreatic cystic neoplasms revisited: part II. Mucinous cystic neoplasms. Surg Oncol 20:93-101
10. Berindoague R, Targarona E, Savelli A et al (2007) Mucinous cystadenocarcinoma of the pancreas diagnosed in postpartum. Langenbecks Arch Surg 392:493-496
11. Herring AA, Graubard MB, Gan SI, Schwaitzberg SD (2007) Mucinous cystadenocarcinoma of the pancreas during pregnancy. Pancreas 34:470-473
12. Wiseman JE, Yamamoto M, Nguyen TD et al (2008) Cystic pancreatic neoplasm in pregnancy: a case report and review of the literature. Arch Surg 143:84-86
13. Tanaka S, Kawamura T, Nakamura N et al (2007) Mucinous cystadenocarcinoma of the pancreas developing during hormone replacement therapy. Dig Dis Sci 52:1326-1328
14. Shimada K, Iwase K, Aono T et al (2009) A case of advanced mucinous cystadenocarcinoma of the pancreas with peritoneal dissemination responding to gemcitabine. Gan To Kagaku Ryoho 36:995-998
15. Mitsuhashi T, Murata N, Sobajima J et al (2001) A case of pseudomyxoma peritonei with a pancreatic cancer treated by the intraperitoneal administration of cisplatinum. Gan To Kagaku Ryoho 28:1670-1673
16. Limmathurotsakul D, Rerknimitr P, Korkij W et al (2007) Metastatic mucinous cystic adenocarcinoma of the pancreas presenting as Sister Mary Joseph's nodule. J Pancreas 8:344-349
17. Wood, D, Silberman AW, Heifetz L et al (1990) Cystadenocarcinoma of the pancreas: neoadjuvant therapy and CEA monitoring. J Surg Oncol 43:56-60
18. Pan ZG, Wang B (2007) Anaplastic carcinoma of the pancreas associated with a mucinous cystic adenocarcinoma. A case report and review of the literature. J Pancreas 8:775-782
19. Sarnaik AA, Saad AG, Mutema GK et al (2003) Osteoclast-like giant cell tumor of the pancreas associated with a mucinous cystadenocarcinoma. Surgery 133:700-701
20. Wu, J, Jiao Y, Dal Molin M et al (2011) Whole-exome sequencing of neoplastic cysts of the pancreas reveals recurrent mutations in components of ubiquitin-dependent pathways. Proc Natl Acad Sci USA 108:21188-21193
21. Wu, J, Matthaei H, Maitra A et al (2011) Recurrent GNAS mutations define an unexpected pathway for pancreatic cyst development. Sci Transl Med 3:92ra66

Part II

Neuroendocrine Pancreatic Neoplasms

Massimo Falconi

Pancreatic neuroendocrine neoplasms (PanNENs) are rare entities, with a wide spectrum of clinical presentations. Affected patients seek medical assistance due to symptoms resulting from either hormonal hypersecretion or mass effects. Thus, PanNENs are clinically defined as functioning or non-functioning, depending on the presence or absence of a syndrome related to inappropriate hormone secretion. In approximately 10–48% of cases, these tumors are not associated with obvious signs or symptoms of hormone hypersecretion. PanNENs differ both biologically and clinically from pancreatic adenocarcinoma since most are characterized by an indolent course and are associated with longer survival. PanNENs are found in 0.5–1.5% of autopsies; their annual incidence in the population is only 5–10 cases per million persons. Consequently, specific treatment recommendations have been traditionally drawn from a few small series or anecdotally, such that the management of PanNENs is still a matter of debate. In particular, it is unclear whether surgery alters their natural progression. The appropriate surgical approach is strictly correlated with the characteristics of the tumor although a widely accepted strategy is still lacking. This is also due to the heterogeneity of these tumors, accounting for their classification according to various clinical-pathological parameters (WHO Classification) and prognostic factors (TNM staging). The clinical behavior of PanNENs varies from benign to low-grade malignant for well-differentiated tumors/carcinomas to high-grade malignant for poorly differentiated carcinomas. The two major categories of well-differentiated and poorly differentiated tumors reflect the distinct phenotypes and genetic backgrounds and thus perhaps also a distinct histogenesis. Surgical options in the treatment strategy vary from a typical pancreatic resection to total pancreatectomy. The former is usually mandatory for large and localized sporadic pan-

M. Falconi (✉)
Department of Surgery and Oncology, "G.B. Rossi" University Hospital, Verona, Italy
and General Surgery Unit, "Sacro Cuore – Don Calabria" Hospital,
Negrar (VR), Italy
e-mail: massimo.falconi@univr.it

P. Pederzoli and C. Bassi (eds.), *Uncommon Pancreatic Neoplasms*,
Updates in Surgery
DOI: 10.1007/978-88-470-2673-5_7, © Springer-Verlag Italia 2013

creatic tumors or in the presence of symptoms. For small and asymptomatic lesions, more conservative surgery (enucleation or central pancreatectomy) is more appropriate. Given the relatively indolent biological behavior of PanNENs, surgery also has a significant role in locally advanced and metastatic forms. In the setting of MEN 1 syndrome or von Hippel Lindau disease, tumor size and possible symptoms should be considered in the evaluation of proper treatment. Despite recent improvements in the classification, diagnosis, and treatment of PanNENs, the relation between pathological and clinical characteristics, type of treatment, and prognosis is only partially understood.

The following chapters focus on all of these aspects of PanNENs, covering important issues ranging from epidemiology to surgery and from pathology to medical targeted and non-targeted treatments. The discussions contained herein are based on surveys of the most recent literature.

Epidemiology and Clinical Presentation

7

Maria Vittoria Davì, Marco Toaiari and Giuseppe Francia

7.1 Epidemiology of Pancreatic Neuroendocrine Neoplasms

Since the description of the first neuroendocrine neoplasm (NEN), published by Oberdorfer at the beginning of the last century [1], the epidemiology of gastroenteropancreatic-NENs (GEP-NENs) has significantly changed, especially over the last decades. In the largest and most recent series of NENs, including those of the GEP type as well as thoracic and unknown primary NENs, a dramatic increase in their age-adjusted incidence in the USA between 1973 and 2004 was reported, from 1.1 to 5.2 per 100,000 inhabitants per year [2]. Many factors are likely to have contributed to this increase, including the improved classification of NENs and the widespread use of endoscopy for cancer screening and of other sensitive imaging procedures such as endoscopy ultrasound (EUS) and computed tomography CT [3].

Regarding pancreatic NENs (PanNENs), in the series of Yao et al. [2] the reported incidence was 0.32 per 100,000 per year, lower than that of lung, ileal, and rectal NENs (1.35, 0.67, and 0.86 per 100,000 respectively). However, the autoptic incidence of PanNENs is greater, at 1.5% per year, indicating that a consistent subgroup of these tumours is under-diagnosed [4].

In a recent Italian survey conducted in 13 referral centers, among 820 patients with NENs, including 63% with GEP-type, 33% with thoracic-type, and 4% with unknown primary origin, a pancreatic origin accounted for 31% of the entire population whereas 50% were GEP-NENs, identifying the pancreas as the most common site of NEN origin [5]. The higher prevalence of pancreatic tumors in this study may have been due to the inclusion of both sporadic and MEN1-NENs.

M.V. Davì (✉)
Department of Internal Medicine, "G.B. Rossi" University Hospital,
Verona, Italy
e-mail: mariavittoria.davi@ospedaleuniverona.it

P. Pederzoli and C. Bassi (eds.), *Uncommon Pancreatic Neoplasms*,
Updates in Surgery
DOI: 10.1007/978-88-470-2673-5_7, © Springer-Verlag Italia 2013

Table 7.1 Biochemical and clinical characteristics of PanNENs

Type of PanNEN	Peptide	Site	Malignancy (%)	MEN1-associated (%)	Clinical manifestation
Insulinoma	Insulin	Pancreas	10	10	Hypoglycemia
Gastrinoma	Gastrin	Pancreas, Duodenum	80	25	ZES (peptic ulcer, diarrhea, epigastric pain)
VIPoma	VIP	Pancreas	80	8.7	Watery diarrhea, hypokalemia, achlorhydria
Glucagonoma	Glucagon PP	Pancreas	60	3	NME, DM, weight loss, anemia, glossitis, thromboembolism
Somatostatinoma	Somatostatin	Pancreas, Duodenum	80	1	DM, steatorrhea, diarrhea, cholelithiasis
Non-functioning	PP	Pancreas	60	20–30	Mass symptoms

ZES, Zollinger-Ellison syndrome; *VIP*, vasoactive intestinal peptide; *NME*, necrolytic migratory erythema; *DM*, diabetes mellitus; *PP*, pancreatic polypeptide.

PanNENs are classified as functioning (F-) and non-functioning (NF-) according to the accompanying presence of a hormonal syndrome (Table 7.1). NF-PanNENs represent the majority, accounting for 30–40% (up to 60-80% in recent series), whereas, among functioning tumors, insulinomas (17%) are the most frequent neoplasm, followed by gastrinomas (15%), VIPomas (2%), glucagonomas (1%), and somatostatinomas (< 1%) [6]. The peak incidence is during the fifth decade of life, with no difference in the distribution between the sexes.

7.2 Inherited PanNENS

PanNENs are usually sporadic, but they can belong to an inherited syndrome, mainly multiple endocrine neoplasia type 1 (MEN1), which is an autosomal dominant syndrome due to a germline mutation in the MEN1 gene, located on chromosome 11q13 [7]. Other classical features of this syndrome are parathyroid and pituitary tumor/hyperplasia. PanNENs are a frequent manifestation in MEN1, are diagnosed a decade earlier than their sporadic counterpart, and are reported as the cause of death in at least one third of MEN1 patients.

The most common PanNENs in MEN1 are non-functioning forms, with a prevalence ranging from 80 to 100%, whereas gastrinomas and insulinomas, the most frequently functioning tumors, occur with a mean prevalence of 54% (range 20–61%) and 18% (range 7–31%) respectively [8]. PanNENs are often multiple and NF-PanNENs can coexist with insulinomas and gastrinomas in the same patient.

In our experience, in 16 out of 31 (52%) patients with PanNENs associated with MEN1, PanNEN was the manifestation that led to the diagnosis of MEN1, since the almost constant presence of hyperparathyroidism is either very often unrecognized or considered sporadic [9]. Thus, if biochemical screening for MEN1 was performed in all patients with PanNENs, an increased number of sporadic PanNENs would be diagnosed as MEN1. Although the prevalence of PanNENs in MEN1 patients has been assessed in several series, the prevalence of MEN1 in PanNENs has not been evaluated, except in the Italian survey, in which the association of NENs with MEN1 occurred in 1 of every 14 patients [5]. Accordingly, clinical and biochemical screening is mandatory in every PanNEN patient in order to determine whether it represents MEN1 syndrome, especially in patients with co-existing primary hyperparathyroidism and/or pituitary adenoma, in the presence of multiple lesions, and/or patients of young age. The clinical suspicion of MEN1 should always be confirmed by a MEN1 mutational analysis. In the event of a positive result, screening can be performed on all relatives and an early diagnosis of the neoplasms made.

The autosomal dominantly inherited von Hippel Lindau (VHL) syndrome is caused by mutations in the VHL gene, located on chromosome 3p25-26. It is associated with PanNENs in 12.3–30% of cases, as well as with other neoplasms, such as renal cell carcinoma, pheochromocytoma, spinal, central nervous system and retinal hemangioblastoma, endolymphatic sac neoplasm, and epididymal cystadenoma [10]. VHL-associated PanNENs are usually non-functioning and can be malignant in 17% of cases, mainly in tumors > 3 cm in size.

Rarely, PanNENs occur as a component of tuberous sclerosis, another genetic disorder.

7.3 Non-functioning Pancreatic NENs

From a clinical point of view, NF-PanNENs are defined as tumors without clinical symptoms arising from hormonal hypersecretion. Small incidental NF-PanNENs are increasingly being recognized because of the more widespread use of new and more sensitive imaging procedures [11]. Most neoplasms ≤ 2 cm are likely to be benign or intermediate-risk lesions and only 6% of these are malignant when incidentally discovered [12].

However, when NF-PanNENs are diagnosed because they have become symptomatic, they are frequently in an advanced stage, with liver metastases. In these cases, the most frequent presenting symptoms are abdominal pain, weight loss, anorexia, and nausea; less frequently, patients present with intra-abdominal hemorrhage, jaundice, or a palpable mass [13]. At first diagnosis, the incidence of liver metastases ranges from 32% to 73%. The median overall survival of patients with NF-PanNENs is 38 months, with a 5-year survival rate of 43%. Factors that are more significantly associated with poor survival are the presence of distant metastases, mainly in liver and bone, and the degree of tumor differentiation [13].

7.4 Insulinoma

Insulinomas are the most common F-PanNENs, with an annual incidence of four cases in one million people. Moreover, these tumors are the most frequent cause of hyperinsulinemic hypoglycemia in adults. Whereas the mean age of patients presenting with sporadic insulinomas is 45 years (range 8–82), MEN1-associated tumors are typically diagnosed at a younger age (25 years or less). A slight female preponderance (female to male ratio 1.4:1) has also been reported [14].

Malignant insulinomas are seen in < 10% of patients and multiple insulinomas in about 10%, most typically in association with MEN1 syndrome. Extrapancreatic localizations (mainly in the ileum, spleen, and duodenal wall) account for < 1% of the cases.

The clinical presentation of insulinoma has changed over the last few years. Although hypoglycemic symptoms usually appear during fasting, postprandial hypoglycemia, previously considered a very uncommon presentation, is increasingly being reported at the time of diagnosis [15]. In fact, in a large series from the Mayo Clinic, post-prandial hypoglycemia was described in 6% of the patients as the only symptom and in 21% it was associated with fasting hypoglycemia [16]. Symptoms of hypoglycemia can generally be classified into two major groups: neuroglycopenic, due to brain glucose deprivation, and neurogenic, due to adrenergic activation. In the first group, dizziness, tiredness, diplopia, headache, blurred vision, mental confusion, abnormal behavior, epilepsy, and coma are seen, while in the second group sweating, trembling, sensation of warmth, anxiety, weakness, nausea, vomiting, and palpitations are characteristic. Insulinoma should be suspected in the presence of Whipple's triad (symptoms or signs consistent with hypoglycemia; glucose level < 50 mg/dl; relief of symptoms after administration of glucose). To confirm the diagnosis, the supervised 72-h fasting test is considered the "gold standard" [17], although in a few cases it can produce negative results, especially in patients with post-prandial symptoms [16]. In 2009, the Endocrine Society's clinical practice guidelines for the management of hypoglycemic disorders established a lower cut-off of insulin of ≥ 3 μU/ml (≥ 18 pmol/l), replacing the previous cut-off of 6 μU/ml (36 pmol/l), in the presence of glycemia < 55 mg/dl, whereas the cut-offs of C-peptide and proinsulin were not modified (respectively, ≥ 0.6 ng/ml or 0.2 nmol/l and ≥ 5 pmol/l). These new criteria were suggested when, at the end of the 1990s, a more sensitive insulin assay became available. Only after the biochemical diagnosis of insulinoma should imaging procedures be performed, with the aim of localizing the tumor as this is of paramount importance in planning the surgical strategy [15].

7.5 Gastrinoma

Zollinger-Ellison Syndrome (ZES) is a rare endocrine disorder (incidence 1–1.5 cases/million/year) caused by ectopic gastrin hypersecretion from duodenal or pancreatic gastrinomas [18]. Gastrinoma is the second most common type of F-PanNEN after insulinoma [11]. In the sporadic form, it occurs most frequently in individuals between the ages of 48 and 55 years and it is slightly more common in males (54–56%). In 20-30% of patients, ZES is part of MEN1 and symptoms occur at an earlier age (32–35 years).

Clinical presentation is characterized by severe peptic ulcer (75–98% of cases), heartburn (44–56%) nausea/vomiting (12–30%), diarrhea (30–75%), gastrointestinal bleeding (44–75%), and weight loss (7–53%) [19-21]. These symptoms correlate with the high gastric acid output due to gastrin hypersecretion. Disease manifestations have changed recently, reflecting the widespread use of proton pump inhibitors (PPIs). These drugs mask the typical symptoms, resulting in a diagnostic delay that could have a negative impact on clinical course and prognosis. In fact, multiple ulcers or ulcers located in unusual sites are seen less frequently than in the past; instead, nowadays, the majority of ZES patients harbor a single typical duodenal ulcer. *Helicobacter pylori* is positive in < 50% of patients. In addition, the resolution of diarrhea following PPI use by patients with duodenal ulcer has been advocated as a criterion suggestive of a ZES diagnosis [22]. Although patients with MEN1 most commonly have parathyroid hyperplasia as the initial manifestation, ZES onset can precede the diagnosis of hyperparathyroidism in 45% of cases [23]. Chronic hypergastrinemia in ZES/MEN1 can stimulate the proliferation of parietal cells and gastric enterochromaffin-like cells, leading to gastric carcinoid (type 2) development. Finally, in 6% of patients with ZES, Cushing's syndrome, due to ectopic ACTH secretion, can complicate the clinical course and worsen the prognosis [18].

In ZES, the primary tumor is located in the duodenum (50–70%) or pancreas (25–40%). Duodenal lesions are even more prevalent in patients with MEN1 (70–90%); these tumors are generally small (< 1 cm) and multifocal. Metastases are very frequent, mainly in patients with pancreatic tumors > 2 cm, and occur firstly in regional lymph nodes and in the liver (70–80% at diagnosis) and later in bones (12%) [1]. The presence of liver metastases has a negative impact on the prognosis and in 25% of patients gastrinoma shows an aggressive behavior, with an overall 10-year survival of 30% [24].

The biochemical diagnosis of ZES requires the demonstration of an inappropriate elevation of serum gastrin in spite of hyperchlorhydria. Accordingly, in these patients autoimmune atrophic gastritis, in which hypergastrinemia is secondary to hypochlorhydria, must be ruled out. Basal gastrin levels elevated > 10-fold, in the presence of gastric pH < 2, is diagnostic of ZES [19]. Since hypochlorhydria induced by PPI is the most frequent cause of high gastrin levels, this class of drugs need to be discontinued at least 1 week before the diagnostic work-up. In these cases, physicians should be aware of the possible complications due to acid hypersecretion. When diagnosis is equivocal, a positive secretin stimulation test, defined as a gastrin increase > 120 pg/ml over the basal level, is considered diagnostic [19].

7.6 VIPoma

The association of refractory diarrhea and hypokalemia was first described by Priest and Alexander [25] and Verner and Morrison [26], in 1957 and 1958, respectively. Only 15 years later, in 1973, the syndrome was correlated with elevated levels of circulating vasoactive intestinal polypeptide 1 (VIP) and VIP-secreting tumor (VIPoma) [27]. VIPoma is a rare tumor, with an annual estimated incidence of 0.1/million individuals [18]. Its prevalence in PanNENs is 0.6–1% (11) and the mean patient age at presentation is 48–51 years [28, 29].

VIP stimulates intestinal and pancreas secretion and inhibits electrolyte and water absorption in the bowel as well as gastric acid secretion. In addition, it induces bone reabsorption, glycogenolysis, and vasodilatation. These effects account for the clinical presentation, which includes watery diarrhea, the most prominent symptom (100%); hypokalemia (< 3 mEq/l), achlorhydria, weight loss (45%), metabolic acidosis, hypercalcemia (50%), carbohydrate intolerance (50%), and flushing (0–33%) [30-32]. Diarrhea is characterized by a large fecal volume that can exceed 6–8 l per day and does not subside after fasting and/or following treatment with antidiarrheal medications. It is intermittent in 53% or continuous in 47% of cases [18]. Marked asthenia, muscular weakness, and cramps are common, striking symptoms and are correlated with hypokalemia. This electrolyte alteration can be so severe (< 2.5 mEq/l) as to cause cardiac rhythm alterations and even sudden death. Hypotension can occur as a consequence of dehydration and vasodilatation. A VIPoma crisis can be life-threatening, with patients requiring intensive care based on treatment with somatostatin analogues, corticosteroids, and aggressive fluid and electrolyte replacement. However, in other cases, VIPomas sometimes present at the onset as NF-PanNENs.

Most VIPomas are sporadic and 70–80% originate from the pancreas, mostly from the tail (50–75%). Other sites are the retroperitoneum, mediastinum, lung, jejunum, and sympathetic ganglia. In 40–70% of patients, the tumors are metastatic at presentation. VIPomas are multifocal in 4% of patients and associated with MEN1 in 8.7% [18].

Regarding tumor characteristics and disease prognosis, Soga et al. (28), in their large series (241 patients), found statistically significant differences between pancreatic vs. extrapancreatic tumors in terms of frequency of an accompanying syndrome (84 vs. 96%), tumor size > 2 cm (79 vs. 100%), rate of metastases (56 vs. 29%), and rate of malignancy (64 vs. 33%). In that study, the 5-year survival rate for patients with pancreatic VIPoma was 69% (60% in patients with metastases vs. 94% in those without metastatic disease). In the

Mayo Clinic series reported by Smith et al., mean survival was 3.6 years, with the longest survival reaching 15 years [31].

The diagnosis is based on the coexistence of compatible symptoms and elevated serum VIP levels (mean levels in three large series were 963, 683, and 698 pg/ml) [29-31]. VIPoma can produce additional peptides, including pancreatic polypeptide, calcitonin, gastric inhibitory peptide, gastrin, glucagon, insulin, somatostatin, growth-hormone-releasing hormone, and peptide histidine methionine (PHM) [30].

7.7 Glucagonoma

Glucagonoma is a very rare F-PanNEN, with an annual estimated incidence of 1/20 million; only 3% of cases are associated with MEN1 syndrome. The so-called glucagonoma syndrome typically consists of necrolytic migratory erythema (NME, 70% of cases), diabetes mellitus (76–94%), weight loss (70-80%), anemia (80%), glossitis (30%), and thromboembolism (10–30%). The etiopathogenesis of NME is largely unknown but is thought to involve a reduction of plasma amino acid concentrations (glutamine and alanine) and hypovitaminosis B as a result of the hyperglucagonemia [33]. Pancreatic polypeptide, which very often is co-secreted in excess in glucagonomas, can play a role in the development of NME and weight loss: in fact, it potentiates the catabolic effects of glucagon by inhibiting food intake and stimulating energy expenditure [34]. High levels of glucagon (> 500 pg/ml, normal value 50–200 pg/ml) are usually associated with the syndrome, whereas a slight elevation (between 200 and 500 pg/ml) is also seen in patients with renal and liver failure, burns, Cushing syndrome, diabetic ketoacidosis, a hyperosmolar non-ketosis state, acute pancreatitis, myocardial infarction, severe infection, and fasting [35]. By the time of diagnosis, almost 60% of patients already have metastases [36].

7.8 Somatostatinoma

Somatostatinoma is a rarer PanNEN than glucagonoma, with an annual incidence of 1 case/40 million. The pancreas is the most common site of somatostatinoma (68%), followed by the duodenal wall (19%), the ampulla of Vater (3%), and the small intestine (3%) [37]. Only 1% of somatostatinomas are associated with MEN1 syndrome, whereas a duodenal localization is found in von Recklinghausen's disease (neurofibromatosis type 1) in up to 50% of cases [38]. Pancreatic somatostatinomas are usually malignant (80%), of large dimension, and present with liver metastases. In rare cases they are associated with a typical syndrome that includes diabetes mellitus (due to the inhibition of insulin release), biliary stasis, and gallstones (due to the inhibition of biliary motility), diarrhea, and steatorrhea (due to alterations in intestinal motility and a reduction of pancreatic enzyme secretion) [39].

References

1. Oberdorfer S (1907) Karzinoide tumoren des Dunndarms. Frankf Z Pathol 1:426-32
2. Yao JC, Hassan M, Phan A et al (2008) One hundred years after "carcinoid": epidemiology of and prognostic factors for neuroendocrine tumors in 35,825 cases in the United States. J Clin Oncol 26:3063-72
3. Rindi G, Bordi C, La Rosa S et al (2011) Gastroenteropancreatic (neuro)endocrine neoplasms: The histology report. Dig Liver Dis 43:356-360
4. Kimura W, Kuroda A, Morioka Y (1991) Clinical pathology of endocrine tumors of the pancreas. Analysis of autopsy cases. Dig Dis Sci 36:933-942
5. Faggiano A, Ferolla P, Grimaldi F et al (2011) Natural history of gastro-enteropancreatic and thoracic neuroendocrine tumors. Data from a large prospective and retrospective Italian Epidemiological Study: The NET MANAGEMENT STUDY. J Endocrinol Invest [Epub ahead of print]
6. Modlin IM, Zikusova M, Kidd M et al (2006) The history and epidemiology of neuroendocrine tumours. In: Caplin M and Kvols L (Eds) Handbook of neuroendocrine tumors, Bioscentifica
7. Brandi ML, Gagel RF, Angeli A et al (2001) Guidelines for diagnosis and therapy of MEN type 1 and type 2. J Clin Endocrinol Metab 86:5658-71
8. Jensen RT, Berna MJ, Bingham DB et al (2008) Inherited pancreatic endocrine tumor syndromes: advances in molecular pathogenesis, diagnosis, management, and controversies. Cancer 1:1807-43
9. Davì MV, Boninsegna L, Dalle Carbonare L et al (2011) Presentation and outcome of pancreaticoduodenal endocrine tumors in multiple endocrine neoplasia type 1 syndrome. Neuroendocrinology 94:58-65
10. Blansfield JA, Choyke L, Morita SY et al (2007) Clinical, genetic and radiographic analysis of 108 patients with von Hippel-Lindau disease (VHL) manifested by pancreatic neuroendocrine neoplasms (PNETs). Surgery 142:814-818
11. Vagefi PA, Razo O, Deshpande V et al (2007) Evolving patterns in the detection and outcomes of pancreatic neuroendocrine neoplasms: the Massachusetts General Hospital experience from 1977 to 2005. Arch Surg 142:347-354
12. Bettini R, Partelli S, Boninsegna L et al (2011) Tumor size correlates with malignancy in nonfunctioning pancreatic endocrine tumor. Surgery 150:75-82
13. Falconi M, Bartsch DK, Eriksson B et al (2012) ENTS Consensus Guidelines for the Management of Patients with Digestive Neuroendocrine Neoplasms of the Digestive System. Welldifferentiated pancreatic non-functioning tumors. Neuroendocrinology 95:120-134
14. Service FJ, McMahon MM, O'Brien PC et al (1991) Functioning insulinoma – incidence, recurrence and long term survival of patient: a 60-year study. Mayo Clinic Proc 66:711-719
15. Davi' MV, Falconi M (2009) Pancreas: Insulinoma--new insights into an old disease. Nat Rev Endocrinol 5:300-302
16. Placzkowski KA, Vella A, Thompson GB et al (2009) Secular trends in the presentation and management of functioning insulinoma at the Mayo Clinic, 1987–2007. J Clin Endocrinol Metab 94:1069-1073
17. Cryer PE, Axelrod L, Grossman AB et al (2009) Evaluation and Management of Adult Hypoglycemic Disorders: An Endocrine Society Clinical Practice Guideline. J Clin Endocrinol Metab 94:709-728
18. Kaltsas GA, Besser GM, Grossman AB (2004) The diagnosis and medical management of advanced neuroendocrine tumors. Endocr Rev 25:458-511
19. Jensen RT, Cadiot G, Brandi ML et al (2012) ENETS Consensus Guidelines for the Management of patients with digestive neuroendocrine neoplasms: functional pancreatic endocrine tumor syndromes. Neuroendocrinology 95:98-119
20. Metz DC, Jensen RT (2008) Gastrointestinal neuroendocrine tumors: pancreatic endocrine tumors. Gastroenterology 135:1469-92
21. Kulke MH, Anthony LB, Bushnell DL et al (2010) NANETS treatment guidelines: well differentiated neuroendocrine tumors of the stomach and pancreas. Pancreas 39:735-752

7 Epidemiology and Clinical Presentation

22. Cadiot G et al (2007) Zollinger-Ellison Syndrome. Unresolved and Controversial Aspects. In: Modlin IM and Oberg K (Eds) A century of advances in neuroendrocrine tumor biology and treatment Felsenstein C.C.C.P, pp 66-74
23. Gibril P, Schumann M, Pace A, Jensen RT (2004) Zollinger Ellison syndrome and multiple endocrine neoplasia type 1 (MEN 1): a prospective NIH study of 107 patients and comparison with 1009 patients from the literature. Medicine 83:43-83
24. Weber HC, Venzon DJ, Lin JT et al (1995) Determinants of metastatic rate and survival in patients with Zollinger-Ellison syndrome: a prospective long-term study. Gastroenterology 108:1637-1649
25. Priest WM, Alexander MK (1957)Islet cell tumor of the pancreas with peptic ulceration, diarrhea and hypokalemia. Lancet 273:1145-1147
26. Verner JV, Morrison AB (1958) Islet cell tumour and a syndrome of refractory watery diarrhea and hypokalemia. Am J Med 25:374-380
27. Bloom SR, Polak JM, Pearse AGE (1973)Vasoactive intestinal peptide and watery –diarrhea syndrome. Lancet 2:14-16
28. Soga J, Yakuwa Y (1998) Vipoma/diarrheogenic syndrome: a statistical evaluation of 241 reported cases. J Exp Clin Cancer Res 17:389-400
29. Peng SY, Li JT, Liu YB et al (2004) Diagnosis and treatment of VIPoma in China: (case report and 31 cases review) diagnosis and treatment of VIPoma Pancreas 28:93-97
30. Ghaferi-Karen AA, Choinacki A Long WD, Cameron JL et al (2008) Pancreatic VIPomas: subject review and one Institutional experience. J Gastrointest Surg 12:382-393
31. Smith SL, Branton SA, Avino AJ et al (1998) Vasoactive intestinal polypeptide secreting islet cell tumors: a 15-year experience and review of the literature. Surgery 124:1050-1055
32. Nikou GC, Toubanakis C, Nikolaou P et al (2005) VIPomas: An update in diagnosis and management in series of 11 patients. Hepatogastroenterology 52:1259-1265
33. van Beek AP, de Haas ERM, van Vloten WA et al (2004) The glucagonoma syndrome and necrolytic migratory erythema: a clinical review. Eur J of Endocrinol 151:531-537
34. Asakawa A, Inui A, Yuzuriha H et al (2003) Characterization of the effects of pancreatic polypeptide in the regulation of energy balance. Gastroenterology 124:1325-1336
35. Wermers RA, Fatourechi V, Wynne AG et al (1996) The glucagonoma syndrome. Clinical and pathologic features in 21 patients. Medicine 75:53-63
36. Hellman P, Andersson M, Rastad J et al (2000) Surgical strategy for large or malignant endocrine pncreatic tumors. World J Surg 24:1353-1360
37. Kimura R, Hayashi Y, Takeuchi T et a (2004). Large duodenal somatostatinoma in the third portion associated with severe glucose intolerance. Intern Med 43:704-707
38. Mao C, Shah A, Hanson DJ et al (1995) Von Recklingausen's disease associated with duodenal somatostatinoma: contrast of duodenal versus pancreatic somatostatinomas. J Surg Oncol 59.67-73
39. Krejs GJ, Orci L, Conlon JM, et al (1979) Somatostatinoma syndrome. Biochemical, morphologic and clinical features. N Engl J Med 301:285-292

Pathology and Genetics

8

Aldo Scarpa and Vincenzo Corbo

8.1 Introduction

Pancreatic endocrine neoplasms (PanNENs) are epithelial tumors affecting adults between the ages of 40 and 60 [1]. They are usually solitary and sporadic but may be part of hereditary syndromes, including multiple endocrine neoplasia type 1 (MEN1), von Hippel Lindau (VHL), neurofibromatosis type 1 (NF1) and tuberous sclerosis complex (TSC).

PanNENs are clinically defined as functioning (F-) or non-functioning (NF-). Patients with F-PanNEN present with a syndrome related to inappropriate hormone secretion. These tumors include insulinomas, gastrinomas, glucagonomas, VIPomas, and somatostatinomas [2-7]. The majority of patients harbor NF-PanNENs and usually present with mass-related symptoms of abdominal pain, nausea, or weight loss. With the exception of insulinomas, most PanNENs, either functional or non-functional, are diagnosed when they have developed into extensive malignant disease, and liver metastases are common. Patients with well-differentiated NF-PanNENs have a 5-year survival rate of approximately 65% and a 10-year survival rate of 45% [3, 8, 9].

8.2 Classification

The 2010 classification of the World Health Organization (WHO) (Table 8.1) identifies two categories based on tumor morphology: well-differentiated neuroendocrine neoplasms (PanNENs) and poorly differentiated neuroendocrine

---

A. Scarpa (✉)
Department of Pathology and Diagnostics, Pathology Unit, "G.B. Rossi"
University Hospital and ARC-NET Research Centre, University of Verona,
Verona, Italy
e-mail: aldo.scarpa@univr.it

P. Pederzoli and C. Bassi (eds.), *Uncommon Pancreatic Neoplasms*,
Updates in Surgery
DOI: 10.1007/978-88-470-2673-5_8, © Springer-Verlag Italia 2013

Table 8.1 World Health Organization classification of PanNEN (from [1])

Well-differentiated neuroendocrine neoplasm (NEN)
NEN G1
NEN G2
Poorly differentiated neuroendocrine carcinoma (NEC)
Large-cell NEC
Small-cell NEC

carcinomas (NECs) [10]. The latter are invariably high-grade malignancies while the former include more than 90% PanNENs with a clinical behavior varying from indolent to malignant, which cannot be predicted based on either tissue architecture or cytological features.

8.3 Pathology

Macroscopically, PanNENs are usually solitary, solid masses, from 1 to 5 cm in diameter, with rounded borders. The expansive pattern of growth determines compression and deviation of the main pancreatic and biliary ducts and of adjacent structures when extending outside the pancreas. The usual PanNEN is rich in small vessels and has scant fibrotic stroma. Necrotic yellowish foci can be observed in larger masses. Features of malignancy evident at macroscopic examination include involvement of the perivisceral fat and invasion of the duodenal wall or adjacent organs. PanNENs may have unusual features, including cystic aspects, and may lead to be misinterpreted as cystic neoplasia; more rarely, they show considerable fibrosis, mimicking ductal adenocarcinoma.

Microscopically, the majority of PanNENs are well-differentiated tumors that grow as solid nests or with trabecular patterns (Fig. 8.1), although glandular, acinar, and cribriform features are observed as well. A rich vascularization is typical. Necrosis can be present as either confluent areas ("infarct-like") in large tumors, or as punctate foci. Cytologically, PanNENs are composed of small to medium-sized cells with a finely granular cytoplasm and round or oval nuclei with salt-and-pepper chromatin. Tumoral infiltration of the duodenum and/or the biliary duct wall together with lymph node metastases identify the malignant forms, as does the involvement of the peripancreatic fat.

Immunohistochemistry serves to confirm the endocrine nature of the neoplasia and thus to differentiate PanNENs from other neoplasms, based on the use of antibodies to at least one general endocrine marker, either synaptophysin [11] or chromogranin A (CgA) [12]. The cytosolic neuron-specific eno-

8 Pathology and Genetics

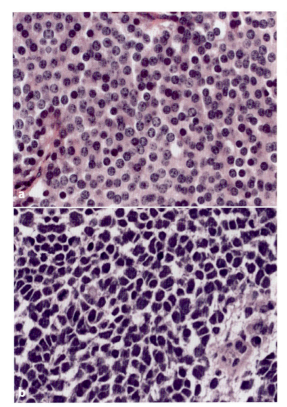

Fig. 8.1 a A typical well-differentiated neuroendocrine neoplasm. **b** A typical poorly differentiated neuroendocrine carcinoma (H&E staining)

lase (NSE) [13] and protein gene product 9.5 (PGP 9.5) [14] are less specific and their diagnostic utility is limited. PanNENs may express the normally produced pancreatic hormones (insulin, glucagon, somatostatin, and pancreatic polypeptide), or hormones of ectopic origin (gastrin, vasoactive intestinal polypeptide, adrenocorticotrophic hormone), or bioamines (serotonin). While any of these may be demonstrated by immunohistochemistry, the information has no clinical application.

Proliferative activity has a recognized prognostic value [10, 15], and its assessment by Ki67 immunostaining is a routine practice in several institutions, including ours (Fig. 8.2).

Poorly differentiated NECs are solid masses with extensive necrosis. Histologically, they resemble small-cell carcinomas or large-cell endocrine carcinomas of others organs, with a high mitotic rate, a proliferative activity of > 20%, and abnormal immunostaining for p53 that correlates with intragenic mutations in the TP53 gene [8, 10, 16]. NECs are usually negative for CgA while synaptophysin persists in the neoplastic cells.

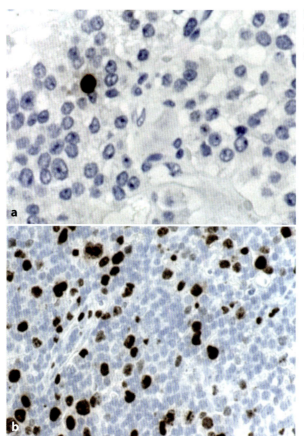

Fig. 8.2 Immunohistochemical staining for Ki67 shows 1% positive cells (a) and 15% positive cells (b)

8.4   Staging and Grading

The European Neuroendocrine Tumor Society (ENETS) has proposed a tumor-node-metastasis (TNM)-based staging system for PanNEN [17] to which subsequent modifications have been proposed [18]. The TNM system is based on the evaluation of the following parameters: size, extrapancreatic invasion, and lymph node and liver metastasis. The clinical need to differentiate between carcinomas at the same stage is facilitated by the use of a grading system based on the measurement of the proliferative activity, by counting mitosis or assessing the immunohistochemical Ki-67 index. Both the TNM staging and the tumor grading systems have been shown to be valid tools for prognostic stratification of PanNENs in clinical practice [19, 20].

8.5 Genetics

Most PanNENs occur sporadically (90%), but they may be part of four hereditary cancer syndromes [9]: Multiple endocrine neoplasia type 1 (MEN1), von Hippel-Lindau disease (VHL), neurofibromatosis type 1 (NF1), and tuberous sclerosis complex (TSC). Of note, studies concerning these familial syndromes have furnished clues as to the molecular mechanisms involved in sporadic PanNEN tumorigenesis. The genetic aberrations associated with PanNENs include chromosomal alterations, epigenetic changes such as methylation, and mutations in single genes. The functional genomic alterations are found at the RNA level and include protein-coding mRNAs and regulatory small RNAs known as "non-coding RNAs" [21].

Accumulating evidence points towards a tumor suppressor pathway and chromatin remodeling as the most important mechanisms associated with PanNENs. Genome-wide analyses by comparative genomic hybridization have shown that virtually all PanNENs display chromosomal alterations [22-24]. Chromosomal losses are slightly more frequent than gains, whereas amplification events are uncommon. The presence of numerous regions of chromosomal losses and gains suggests the existence of two molecular subgroups: one showing frequent allelic imbalances (AI) and another showing low AI [25, 26]. These two subgroups have been shown to correspond to aneuploid and near-diploid tumors, respectively, and their identification was suggested to have prognostic value [26]. The total number of genomic changes per tumor appears to be associated with both tumor burden and disease stage, suggesting the accumulation of genetic alterations during tumor progression. A strong correlation has been found between sex-chromosome loss and an aggressive behavior of PanNENs, namely, the presence of local invasion or metastasis [27]. Retinoblastoma and TP53 gene defects have never been observed in PanNENs but are consistently present in NECs [16]. DNA methylation of the *RASSF1A* gene has been suggested as a major event in PanNENs [28, 29], possibly leading to gene inactivation. However, a very recent study demonstrated RASSF1A expression in the presence of promoter methylation [30]. Mutations in oncogenes are never or rarely observed in PanNENs [31, 32]. Instead, mutations in tumor suppressor genes represent the major genetic anomaly encountered in this type of tumor. Indeed, mutations in the tumor suppressor gene *MEN1* are the most common anomaly associated with PanNENs [33, 34]. *MEN1* encodes for the scaffold protein menin, which is known to interact with several proteins involved in, for example, transcription regulation, maintaince of genome stability, and histone modification.

A recent systematic whole-exome analysis exploiting next-generation sequencing technologies confirmed that MEN1 gene mutations are the most relevant anomalies in PanNEN [32]. More interestingly, mutually exclusive mutations were found in genes involved in chromatin remodeling (*ATRX* and *DAXX*). The majority of the mutations in these genes were associated with the loss of corresponding proteins that normally associate to form a macromolecular complex. This complex is involved in the deposition of histone H3 family member H3.3 at transcriptionally silent regions of the genome, including telomeres, and therefore is responsible for correct nucleosome assembly, the dysfunction of which likely leads to increased DNA damage and genome instability. Furthermore, the loss of ATRX/DAXX seems to be associated with ALT (alternative telomere lengthening), a crucial mechanism by which PanNENs maintain telomere length [35].

In addition to alterations in chromatin-associated genes, other tumor suppressor genes that have been found mutated in PanNENs are *PTEN* and *TSC2*, which are negative regulators of the mTOR pathway. Activation of mTOR pathways in primitive PanNENs was already demonstrated in analyses of expression profiles, which revealed the down-regulation of the *TSC2* gene and alteration of TSC2 and PTEN protein expression in the vast majority of tumors analyzed [36].

Finally, global microRNA expression analysis revealed that the overexpression of a specific microRNA (miR-21) is strongly associated with an aggressive clinical behavior of PanNENs [37]. MicroRNAs are small non-coding RNAs that regulate gene expression by targeting specific mRNAs for degradation or translation inhibition. MiR-21 has several targets, including *PTEN*, whose expression is therefore reduced following up-regulation of the microRNA, leading to mTOR activation as well.

8.6   Conclusions

In patients with PanNENs, the pathology report must include information permitting disease classification, staging, and grading in order to obtain a prognostic evaluation. Genes involved in sporadic PanNEN tumorigenesis mainly belong to tumor suppressor pathways that are responsible for chromatin remodeling and the maintenance of genome stability. The direct consequences of these defective pathways are consistent chromosomal alterations that are a hallmark of PanNENs. Finally, global expression profiling analysis has furnished a strong rationale for the use of targeted therapy in the treatment of advanced-stage disease.

References

1. Klimstra D, Arnold R, Capella C et al (2010) Neuroendocrine neoplasms of the pancreas. In: Bosman F, Carneiro F, Hruban R, et al (eds) World Health Organization classification of tumors of the digestive system. IARC, Lyon
2. O'Toole D, Salazar R, Falconi M et al (2006) Rare functioning pancreatic endocrine tumors. Neuroendocrinology 84:189-195
3. Kloppel G, Rindi G, Anlauf M et al (2007) Site-specific biology and pathology of gastroenteropancreatic neuroendocrine tumors. Virchows Arch 451 Suppl 1:S9-27

8 Pathology and Genetics

4. Jensen RT, Niederle B, Mitry E et al (2006) Gastrinoma (duodenal and pancreatic). Neuroendocrinology 84:173-182
5. de Herder WW, Niederle B, Scoazec JY et al (2006) Well-differentiated pancreatic tumor/carcinoma: insulinoma. Neuroendocrinology 84:183-188
6. Anlauf M, Garbrecht N, Henopp T et al (2006) Sporadic versus hereditary gastrinomas of the duodenum and pancreas: distinct clinico-pathological and epidemiological features. World J Gastroenterol 12:5440-5446
7. Alexakis N, Neoptolemos JP (2008) Pancreatic neuroendocrine tumours. Best Pract Res Clin Gastroenterol 22:183-205
8. Hruban RU, Bishop Pitman M, Klimstra DL (2007) Endocrine Neoplasms, in Silverberg SG, Sobin LH (eds): Tumors of the pancreas. Washington, Armed Forces Institute of Pathology
9. Capelli P, Martignoni G, Pedica F et al (2009) Endocrine neoplasms of the pancreas: pathologic and genetic features. Arch Pathol Lab Med 133:350-364
10. Heitz PU, Komminoth P, Perren A et al (2004) Pancreatic endocrine tumours, in DeLellis RA, Lloyd RV, Heitz PU, et al (eds): World Health Organization Classification of Tumors. Pathology and Genetics of Tumors of Endocrine Organs. IARC Press, Lyon
11. Wiedenmann B, Franke WW, Kuhn C, et al (1986) Synaptophysin: a marker protein for neuroendocrine cells and neoplasms. Proc Natl Acad Sci U S A 83:3500-3504
12. Lloyd RV, Mervak T, Schmidt K et al (1984) Immunohistochemical detection of chromogranin and neuron-specific enolase in pancreatic endocrine neoplasms. Am J Surg Pathol 8:607-14
13. Bishop AE, Polak JM, Facer P et al (1982) Neuron specific enolase: a common marker for the endocrine cells and innervation of the gut and pancreas. Gastroenterology 83:902-15
14. Rode J, Dhillon AP, Doran JF et al (1985) PGP 9.5, a new marker for human neuroendocrine tumours. Histopathology 9:147-158
15. Pelosi G, Bresaola E, Bogina G et al (1996) Endocrine tumors of the pancreas: Ki-67 immunoreactivity on paraffin sections is an independent predictor for malignancy: a comparative study with proliferating-cell nuclear antigen and progesterone receptor protein immunostaining, mitotic index, and other clinicopathologic variables. Hum Pathol 27:1124-1134
16. Yachida S, Vakiani E, White CM et al (2012) Small cell and large cell neuroendocrine carcinomas of the pancreas are genetically similar and distinct from well-differentiated pancreatic neuroendocrine tumors. Am J Surg Pathol 36:173-184
17. Rindi G, Kloppel G, Alhman H et al (2006) TNM staging of foregut (neuro)endocrine tumors: a consensus proposal including a grading system. Virchows Arch 449:395-401
18. Scarpa A, Mantovani W, Capelli P et al (2010) Pancreatic endocrine tumors: improved TNM staging and histopathological grading permit a clinically efficient prognostic stratification of patients. Mod Pathol 23:824-833
19. Fischer L, Kleeff J, Esposito I et al (2008) Clinical outcome and long-term survival in 118 consecutive patients with neuroendocrine tumours of the pancreas. Br J Surg 95:627-635
20. Pape UF, Jann H, Muller-Nordhorn J et al (2008) Prognostic relevance of a novel TNM classification system for upper gastroenteropancreatic neuroendocrine tumors. Cancer 113:256-265
21. Barbarotto E, Schmittgen TD, Calin GA (2008): MicroRNAs and cancer: profile, profile, profile. Int J Cancer 122:969-977
22. Stumpf E, Aalto Y, Hoog A et al (2000) Chromosomal alterations in human pancreatic endocrine tumors. Genes Chromosomes Cancer 29:83-87
23. Speel EJ, Richter J, Moch H et al (1999) Genetic differences in endocrine pancreatic tumor subtypes detected by comparative genomic hybridization. Am J Pathol 155:1787-1794
24. Hu W, Feng Z, Modica I et al (2010) Gene Amplifications in Well-Differentiated Pancreatic Neuroendocrine Tumors Inactivate the p53 Pathway. Genes Cancer 1:360-368
25. Nagano Y, Kim do H, Zhang L et al (2007) Allelic alterations in pancreatic endocrine tumors identified by genome-wide single nucleotide polymorphism analysis. Endocr Relat Cancer 14:483-492
26. Rigaud G, Missiaglia E, Moore PS et al (2001) High resolution allelotype of nonfunctional pancreatic endocrine tumors: identification of two molecular subgroups with clinical implications. Cancer Res 61:285-292

27. Missiaglia E, Moore PS, Williamson J et al (2002) Sex chromosome anomalies in pancreatic endocrine tumors. Int J Cancer 98:532-538
28. Arnold CN, Sosnowski A, Schmitt-Graff A et al (2007) Analysis of molecular pathways in sporadic neuroendocrine tumors of the gastro-entero-pancreatic system. Int J Cancer 120:2157-2164
29. House MG, Herman JG, Guo MZ et al (2003) Aberrant hypermethylation of tumor suppressor genes in pancreatic endocrine neoplasms. Ann Surg 238:423-431; discussion 431-432
30. Malpeli G, Amato E, Dandrea M et al (2011) Methylation-associated down-regulation of RASSF1A and up-regulation of RASSF1C in pancreatic endocrine tumors. BMC Cancer 11:351
31. Corbo V, Beghelli S, Bersani S et al (2012) Pancreatic endocrine tumours: mutational and immunohistochemical survey of protein kinases reveals alterations in targetable kinases in cancer cell lines and rare primaries. Ann Oncol 23:127-134
32. Jiao Y, Shi C, Edil BH et al (2011) DAXX/ATRX, MEN1, and mTOR pathway genes are frequently altered in pancreatic neuroendocrine tumors. Science 331:1199-1203
33. Moore PS, Missiaglia E, Antonello D et al (2001) Role of disease-causing genes in sporadic pancreatic endocrine tumors: MEN1 and VHL. Genes Chromosomes Cancer 32:177-181
34. Corbo V, Dalai I, Scardoni M et al (2010) MEN1 in pancreatic endocrine tumors: analysis of gene and protein status in 169 sporadic neoplasms reveals alterations in the vast majority of cases. Endocr Relat Cancer 17:771-783
35. Heaphy CM, de Wilde RF, Jiao Y et al (2011) Altered telomeres in tumors with ATRX and DAXX mutations. Science 333:425
36. Missiaglia E, Dalai I, Barbi S et al (2010) Pancreatic endocrine tumors: expression profiling evidences a role for AKT-mTOR pathway. J Clin Oncol 28:245-255
37. Roldo C, Missiaglia E, Hagan JP et al (2006) MicroRNA expression abnormalities in pancreatic endocrine and acinar tumors are associated with distinctive pathologic features and clinical behavior. J Clin Oncol 24:4677-4684

Imaging

9

Roberto Pozzi Mucelli, Giovanni Foti and Luigi Romano

9.1 Introduction

Pancreatic neuroendocrine neoplasms (PanNENs) are a heterogeneous group of rare tumors of the pancreas originating from totipotential stem cells or differentiated mature endocrine cells within the exocrine gland. [1] Although rare, occurring in fewer than 1 in 100,000 people per year [2, 3], the frequency of PanNENs is progressively increasing as a result of better awareness by clinicians, radiologists, and pathologists [2].

These neoplasms usually occur sporadically but can occasionally be associated with genetic syndromes, such as multiple endocrine neoplasia type 1 (MEN1), von Hippel–Lindau disease, neurofibromatosis type 1, and tuberous sclerosis [4].

PanNENs produce and secrete hormones to a variable degree. When they produce symptoms related to excessive hormone production, the tumors are classified as syndromic or functioning pancreatic endocrine neoplasms (F-PanNENs) [5].

F-PanNENs are classified according to the name of the predominant hormone they secrete [5]. The two most common F-PanNENs are insulinoma and gastrinoma, followed by VIPoma, glucagonoma, somatostatinoma, and carcinoids [5].

In F-PanNENs, the role of imaging is mainly to detect the tumor [6, 7], which is usually quite small at diagnosis. Imaging also verifies lesion number and location and determines the exact location of the neoplasm, within and/or outside of the pancreas (in tumors with ectopic locations).

R. Pozzi Mucelli (✉)
Department of Pathology and Diagnostics, Radiology Unit, "G.B. Rossi" University Hospital, Verona, Italy
e-mail: roberto.pozzimucelli@univr.it

P. Pederzoli and C. Bassi (eds.), *Uncommon Pancreatic Neoplasms*,
Updates in Surgery
DOI: 10.1007/978-88-470-2673-5_9, © Springer-Verlag Italia 2013

Non-functioning pancreatic endocrine neoplasms (NF-PanNENs) comprise about two-thirds of PanNENs (range: 10–48%), and more than half of all NF-PanNENs are malignant [5, 8-13]. They tend to manifest late, as large masses causing compression symptoms, or may be detected incidentally in asymptomatic patients. The role of imaging studies is to characterize the tumor, differentiating it from other tumor entities and in particular from ductal adenocarcinoma. This is an important distinction because malignant NF-panNENs have a more favorable prognosis (5-year survival rate 40% vs. 3%–5% for adenocarcinoma) [11, 12].

As they are often malignant [14,] NF-PanNENs also require accurate staging and appropriate follow-up.

Multiple imaging techniques have been employed in the evaluation of PanNENs, including ultrasonography (US), computed tomography (CT), and magnetic resonance imaging (MRI). Here we describe the imaging techniques available for the assessment of these rare lesions, pointing out the specific features of each imaging tool.

Also, the typical and atypical imaging features and diagnostic strategies available for both F-PanNENs and NF-PanNENs are analyzed.

9.2 Ultrasound

9.2.1 Imaging Technique

Trans-abdominal US represents a low cost, widely available imaging tool for evaluating PanNENs [15]. However, it does not allow lesion characterization, and correct interpretation of imaging strictly depends on the expertise and skills of the radiologist performing these procedures. Such limitations obviously become significant only in cases in which the pancreatic lesion is small or when an appropriate differential diagnosis is needed.

Also, trans-abdominal US may be diagnostically limited if either the patient's body habitus or gas in the bowel prevents a complete examination of the pancreas [16].

Recently published studies have shown that contrast-enhanced ultrasound (CEUS) can improve the identification of small F-PanNENs and the characterization of NF-PanNENs [17-20]. The intravenously injected contrast material (Sonovue, Bracco, Milan, Italy), together with the possibility to continuously visualize the lesion, allows a dedicated study to be performed, with depiction of the typical hypervascular enhancement pattern shown by the majority of PanNENs [17-20].

Endoscopic ultrasound (EUS) of the pancreas uses a high-frequency probe to generate images of the various regions of the pancreas [21]. Also, if a mass is present, biopsies can be performed through a conventional endoscope [22]. Patients undergoing EUS should fast starting at midnight of the night before the procedure. Intravenous access is established, and the patient is sedated.

After a preliminary endoscopic examination of the upper gastrointestinal tract, an endo-sonographic scope with a water-filled balloon in place is advanced as far into the duodenum as possible, and the duodenum, ampulla, and pancreas are visualized. Difficulty can be encountered if peristalsis is excessive or because of poor patient compliance.

Intraoperative ultrasound (IOUS) takes advantage of the direct placement of the US probe very close to the area of interest. Thus, because of the short distance of the probe to the target, e.g., the pancreas, a high-frequency transducer (7.5 or 10 MHz) can be used, yielding images with greater spatial resolution [23].

During IOUS of the exposed pancreas, the head of the gland is mobilized and the lesser sac is opened. The peritoneal cavity can be filled with warm saline. The transducer is enclosed in a sterile sheath and the pancreas is evaluated along its transverse and longitudinal planes, which permits visualization of both deep and superficial lesions [23, 24]. IOUS can be used to confirm the location of lesions identified preoperatively and to detect small lesions missed on other imaging studies.

9.2.2 Imaging Findings

Commonly, at trans-abdominal US the texture of the pancreatic gland can be considered as comparable to that of the liver. Pancreatic parenchyma is usually relatively hypoechoic in younger patients. An increase of fibrous and/or fatty tissues within the pancreas is usually associated with a relative increase in echogenicity compared to normal liver.

When detectable, small PanNENs (either functioning or non-functioning) appear as well-circumscribed nodules embedded in the pancreatic gland. These lesions are clearly hypoechoic compared to the normal pancreatic parenchyma [15, 17]. The majority of small lesions, measuring < 3 cm in diameter, are usually quite homogeneous on unenhanced US [17]. Small iso-echoic lesions represent an important limitation for this imaging tool since they are frequently missed, especially in younger patients, because of the relatively hypoechoic appearance of the normal gland (Fig 9.1c).

At CEUS, PanNENs typically show early intense enhancement, indicative of hypervascular oval-shaped nodules distinct from the surrounding tissues (Fig. 9.1b, d) [17-20, 25].

Trans-abdominal US usually permits the correct identification of large PanNENs. The majority of these tumors appear as inhomogeneous hypo-/isoechoic masses relative to the normal pancreatic and liver parenchyma (Fig. 9.2) [25]. Most NF-PanNENs are large at presentation, with a well-defined multi-lobulated border and a compressive rather than an infiltrative pattern of growth [20, 25].

NF-PanNENs cannot be reliably characterized using conventional US. (Figs. 9.1, 9.2); however, once they are detected on baseline scan, CEUS

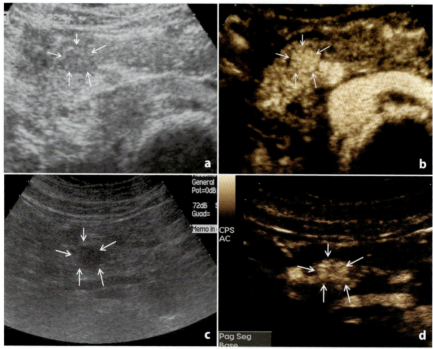

Fig. 9.1 Trans-abdominal US and CEUS imaging findings of small PanNENs. Small iso-echoic tumor (*arrows*) located on the pancreatic head (**a**), showing early intense enhancement (*arrows*) on CEUS (**b**). Typical small hypoechoic insulinoma of the pancreatic head (*arrows* in **c**), seen as a hypervascular focal lesion (*arrows*); for comparison, normal parenchyma as seen on CEUS (**d**)

allows for their dynamic evaluation and characterization. The early and intense enhancement and the slow washout of hypervascularized tumors can be documented (Figs. 9.1, 9.2) and is a key feature in the differential diagnosis with adenocarcinoma, which usually appears as a hypovascular mass [20, 25].

Small lesions, measuring < 3 cm in diameter, usually enhance homogenously [17].

Intralesional necrosis and or hemorrhagic areas, frequently encountered in large lesions, result in inhomogeneous central hypoechoic areas better depicted at CEUS [15, 20, 25].

Large lesions may be associated with the encasement of arterial or venous vessels and with peri-tumoral lymphadenopathy.

Metastatic disease in the liver occurs in about 30% of cases [13, 25] and represents a clear sign of malignancy. The US appearance of the liver metastases is variable. Hyperechoic nodules or a target-like appearances at baseline

9 Imaging

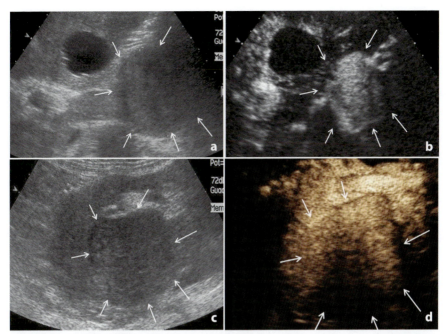

Fig. 9.2 Trans-abdominal US and CEUS imaging findings of NF-PanNENs. A large hypoechoic tumor (*arrows*) located on the pancreatic body (**a**), showing early intense enhancement (*arrows*) on CEUS (**b**). Large well-defined hypoechoic NF-PanNEN of the pancreatic head (*arrows* in **c**), seen as a hypervascular focal lesion (*arrows*) at CEUS (**d**)

US suggests an endocrine nature of the primary tumor, but this pattern is not specific. In other cases, the metastases show a non-specific hypoechoic pattern [15, 25]. A dedicated CEUS study of a suspected liver lesion may point out the typical hypervascularity shown by endocrine tumors during their early dynamic study (Fig. 9.3).

EUS visualizes islet-cell tumors as a relatively hypoechoic area compared with the adjacent pancreas, with smooth and at times slightly irregular margins that are well demarcated.

In the identification of small lesions located in the pancreatic head, EUS has high sensitivity but it may be limited in completely evaluating the tail of the pancreas, depending on its location [26]. A recently published study demonstrated the value of EUS in the preoperative assessment of patients with MEN1 [27].

In the identification of small F-PanNENs during surgery, a combination of intraoperative palpation and IOUS was found to achieve the best results due to the complementary nature of these two techniques.

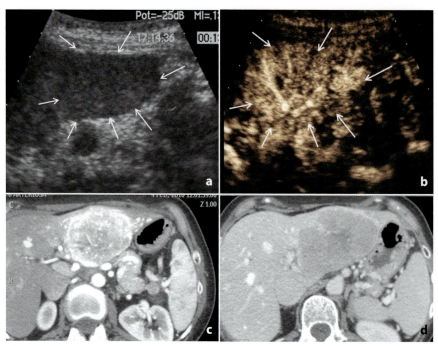

Fig. 9.3 Large liver metastasis from a NF-PanNEN/C studied using trans-abdominal US and CEUS and MDCT. A large, slightly hypoechoic, focal liver lesion (*arrows*) can be appreciated in the left lobe (**a**). The lesion shows early intense enhancement (*arrows*) on CEUS (**b**). At MDCT, during arterial pancreatic phase (**c**), the lesion has the typical hypervascular pattern of endocrine tumors, with subsequent washout during portal venous phase (**d**)

9.3 Computed Tomography

9.3.1 Imaging Technique

Multidetector computed tomography (MDCT) is a widely available imaging technique capable of providing, in a short examination time, images characterized by excellent spatial and contrast resolution. The MDCT protocol should include both unenhanced and enhanced scans, as the former, obtained at baseline, can be useful in the detection of intralesional calcifications (which may occur in F- and NF-PanNENs) (Fig. 9.4), and to accurately plan the dynamic contrast-enhanced study.

The intravenous administration of iodinated contrast agent is needed to optimally visualize the pancreatic parenchyma, increasing contrast resolution [28].

PanNENs are frequently hypervascular focal lesions, appearing as high-attenuating lesions during early contrast-enhancement phases [29, 30] (Figs. 9.5, 9.6). Accordingly, the protocol should include at least two contrast-enhanced phases

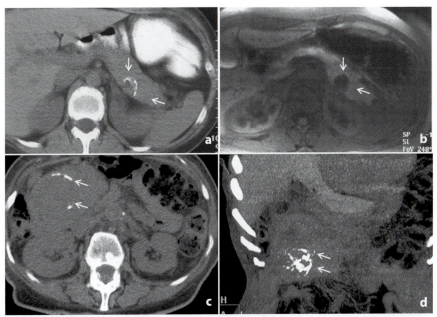

Fig. 9.4 Calcification in PanNENs. Unenhanced CT scan points out a tiny F-PanNEN located in the pancreatic tail, with intralesional calcifications (**a**). These are not depicted on T1-weighted MRI (**b**). A large NF-PanNEN located in the pancreatic head, with intralesional calcifications depicted on unenhanced axial (**c**) and coronal (**d**) scans

[30-32], acquired, respectively, with a 40- to 45-s delay (arterial pancreatic phase) and a 70- to 80-s delay (portal venous phase) after the administration of contrast material (calculated by using the bolus-tracking technique).

However, about 30% of these tumors will have an atypical vascular pattern, resulting in iso- or even hypoattenuating lesions with respect to adjacent pancreatic parenchyma (Fig. 9.7) [13].

In our experience, in most cases the best enhancement is obtained during the arterial pancreatic phase [13]; nonetheless, additional contrast-enhanced scans should be taken in selected cases. An early arterial phase, acquired with a delay of 20–25 s (vascular arterial phase), may be useful in the detection of small tumors characterized by subtle brief enhancement. In addition, it may allow detailed arterial vascular mapping, which is useful for staging locally advanced tumors and for treatment planning (Fig. 9.8).

A late venous phase, acquired with a delay of about 120 s, may be useful for depicting a delayed hypervascular enhancing pattern. A multi-phase imaging protocol therefore offers the advantage of increasing the possibility of demonstrating the typical hypervascular pattern of PanNENs, to allow locoregional staging and the detection of liver metastases [13].

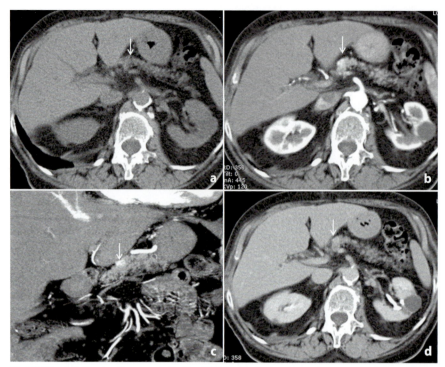

Fig. 9.5 Typical tiny insulinoma studied by MDCT. The lesion (*arrow*) appears isodense on baseline unenhanced scan (**a**). During a contrast-enhanced study, the lesion (*arrow*) shows the typical hyperdensity on axial (**b**) and para-coronal reconstructed images obtained from the arterial pancreatic phase (**c**), showing washout during the venous phase (**d**)

Curvilinear reconstructions should be used to highlight the relationship between primary tumors and the pancreatic and biliary ductal systems (Fig. 9.9).

The patient can be administered a glass of water immediately before the examination, to assure optimal filling of the stomach and duodenum with a low-contrast medium and for better definition of the gastric and duodenal wall. We usually avoid administrating oral iodinated contrast material, to avoid the misinterpretation or masking of hypervascular lesions ectopically located within the duodenal or small-bowel wall.

9.3.2 Imaging Findings

Baseline CT usually depicts PanNENs as isodense masses with respect to normal parenchyma (Figs. 9.5a, 6a, 7a). Thus, the tumor might be missed on an unenhanced scan, unless it has a large diameter and/or is associated with a distorted morphology of the gland [13].

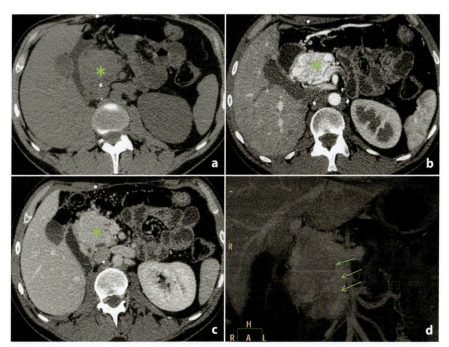

Fig. 9.6 Typical enhancement pattern of NF-PanNEN/Cs studied by MDCT. The lesion (*star*) appears isodense on baseline unenhanced scan (**a**). During contrast-enhanced study, the tumor (*star*) shows the typical hyperdensity on axial images obtained during arterial pancreatic (**b**) and portal venous phases (**c**). Para-coronal reconstructed images obtained during the portal venous phase better depicts encasement of the superior mesenteric vein (*arrows* in **d**)

Tumor inhomogeneity may be caused by globular or lamellar calcifications, seen both in F-panNENs (mostly insulinomas) and in NF-PanNENs, in these cases often associated with large areas of necrosis (Fig. 9.4a, b, d) [33].

During dynamic contrast-enhanced study, both functioning and non-functioning PanNENs usually appear as well-defined round or oval-shaped hypervascular masses [33]. At MDCT, the most frequent peak-enhancement phase is the arterial pancreatic phase whereas rapid washout is frequently seen in the portal venous and late venous phases (Fig. 9.6).

Achieving an intense enhancement is also useful to better define the dimensions of the tumors and to evaluate the relationship with adjacent structures [34] (Fig. 9.10).

Enhancement is usually homogeneous in small lesions, measuring < 3 cm in diameter [13, 33]. Conversely, large tumors, measuring > 3 cm in diameter, are typically inhomogeneous because of the presence of intralesional necrotic areas or cystic degeneration [13, 35], appearing as hypodense areas compared with the viable hypervascularized neoplastic tissue (Fig. 9.9).

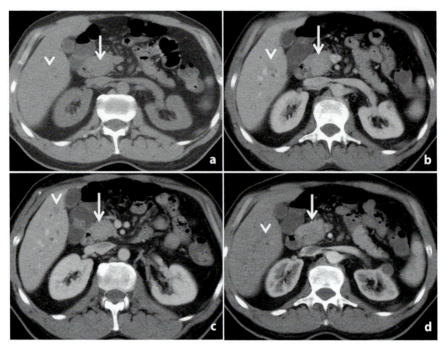

Fig. 9.7 Atypical enhancement pattern of PanNEN/Cs studied by MDCT. The lesion (*arrow*) appears isodense on baseline unenhanced scan (**a**). During contrast-enhanced study, the tumor (*arrow*) is isodense on axial images obtained during arterial pancreatic (**b**) and portal venous phases (**c, d**). Multiple, tiny, slightly hypodense liver metastases are seen in segments V and VI (*arrowhead*)

MDCT, due to its high spatial, contrast, and temporal resolution, is advantageous in loco-regional staging, depicting the encasement of both the arterial (superior mesenteric artery or the celiac axis) and venous (superior mesenteric vein and portal vein) vessels [13, 33]. Three-dimensional reconstruction of the peri-pancreatic vessels may be of help in treatment planning (Fig 9.8).

Neoplastic thrombus within the peri-pancreatic veins has the same density as the mass from which it derives, thus displaying a slightly lower density than the vascular lumen.

Secondary phenomena, such as bile duct dilation or vascular encasement, may be well-demonstrated by means of MDCT, using axial native images and multi-planar dedicated reconstructions (Fig. 9.9b) [13]. Also, dilatation of the biliary tree may be depicted in case of tumors located in the pancreatic head.

Depending on its location, the primary tumor may dislocate or compress adjacent structures such as the stomach and duodenum, spleen and left kidney, and the adrenal gland (Fig. 9.11). Frank invasion into adjacent viscera is rare and is usually associated with the presence of an endocrine carcinoma.

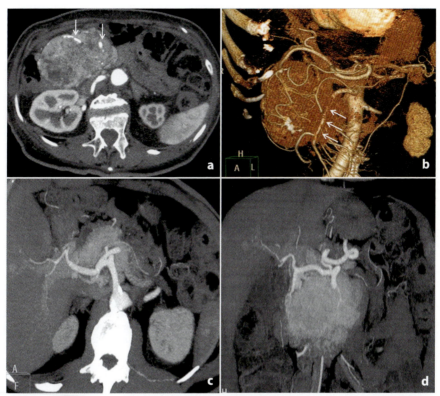

Fig. 9.8 Vascular encasement demonstrated using MDCT reconstructions. A large inhomogeneous NF-PanNEN/C of the pancreatic head is associated with complete encasement of multiple vessels (*arrows*), depicted on axial images. The volume-rendering reconstructed image obtained from the arterial pancreatic dataset (**b**) clearly shows the encasement of multiple vessels, including the superior mesenteric artery (*arrows*). Maximum-intensity projection (MIP) reconstructions (**c, d**) in another patient show involvement of the celiac axis

Even if less accurate than MRI in identifying liver metastases, MDCT represents a reliable tool for the identification of metastatic involvement of the liver in case of PanNENs [13, 33].

There is no difference between the metastases of F-PanNENs and NF-PanNENs. These lesions usually share imaging features of primary tumors, i.e., slightly hypodense compared with the normal parenchyma on unenhanced CT scan, and hyperdense hypervascular lesions (sometimes with a target-like pattern) on arterial enhanced scan [30, 36]. Liver metastases typically show washout during portal venous and late venous phases, resulting in lesions hypodense to normal liver parenchyma (Fig. 9.3c, d). Calcifications may be present as well.

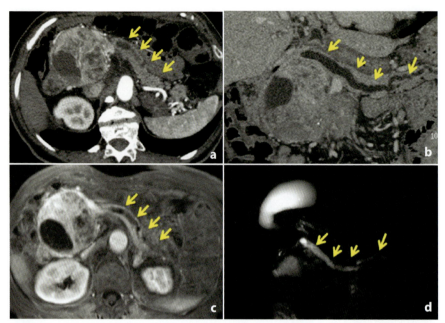

Fig. 9.9 Involvement of the main pancreatic duct, demonstrated using MDCT and MRI. A large inhomogeneous NF-PanNEN/C of the pancreatic head is associated with the complete upstream dilatation of the main pancreatic duct (*arrows* in **a**). The dilatation is better depicted using curvilinear reconstruction in the para-coronal plane (**b**). Dilatation of the main pancreatic duct (*arrows*) is well-depicted using contrast enhanced MRI, as seen on the axial plane (**c**) and on the MRCP image (**d**)

Hypovascular liver metastases may be associated with hypovascular primary tumors (Fig. 9.7).

The typical features of NF-PanNENs, such as a well-demarcated hypervascular mass with a compressive pattern of growth, are present in about 70% of patients [13, 15, 28, 33]. In the other 30%, the pattern is non-specific and a reliable differential diagnosis with ductal adenocarcinoma is not possible [37], since the tumor is mainly hypodense compared with the pancreatic parenchyma (Fig. 9.7).

When the mass is large and well-circumscribed, a ductal adenocarcinoma can be excluded, but the problem of differential diagnosis from other rare, solid tumors remains, including solid variants of micro-cystic cystadenoma and pancreatic metastases.

PanNENs may appear as iso-attenuating to normal pancreas in pancreatic phase CT images, and sometimes are better delineated in the portal venous phase [13, 38]. Late enhancement of the tumor may be explained by extensive necrosis, resulting in a slower washout from the mass, due to the reduced vascularization [39].

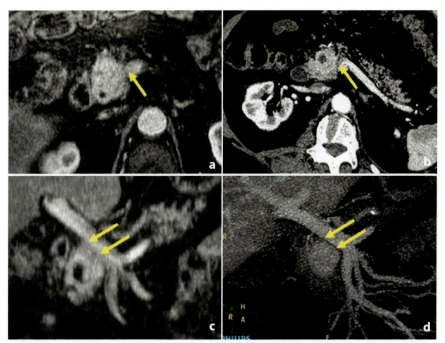

Fig. 9.10 Involvement of peri-tumoral vessels, assessed using MDCT and MRI. A relatively small but inhomogeneous NF-PanNEN/C of the pancreatic head is located close to the superior mesenteric vein (*arrow*) on axial portal-enhanced MRI (**a**) and MDCT (**b**). Coronal reconstructions obtained using MRI (**c**) do not rule out vessel, involvement (*arrows*). Conversely, MDCT (**d**), with its higher spatial resolution, demonstrates the presence of an adipose interface between tumor and vessel (*arrows*)

9.4 Magnetic Resonance Imaging

9.4.1 Imaging Technique

In patients with PanNENs, the information obtained with MRI is similar to that obtained with CT, with the additional advantage that the patient is spared radiation exposure. However, due to its relatively limited availability and the longer examination time, MRI is not as widely used as CT for imaging pancreatic tumors.

State-of-the-art MRI of pancreatic neoplasms is optimally performed with 1.5 Tesla gradient systems using phased-array coils to improve the signal-to-noise ratio, optimized with thin slices and a small field of view [13, 40]. Breath-hold acquisitions are obtained with fast spin echo (FSE) or gradient echo (GRE) sequences and echo planar imaging. A moderately T2-weighted FSE and single-shot FSE (SSFSE) should be obtained, followed by T1-weighted in-phase GRE and T1-weighted opposed-phase GRE.

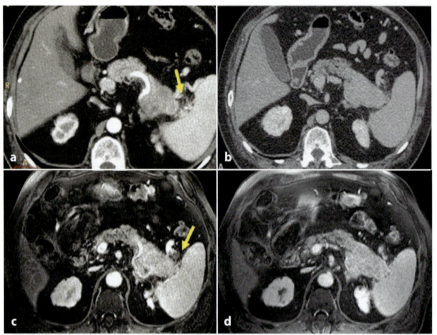

Fig. 9.11 Infiltration of adjacent structures as assessed using MDCT (**a**, **b**) and MRI (**c**, **d**). A large inhomogeneous NF-PanNEN/C of the pancreatic tail infiltrates the splenic hilum and peri-pancreatic fat (*arrow*), as well-depicted with both modalities

T1-weighted images with fat suppression have proven to be useful for imaging the pancreatic gland, allowing high contrast resolution between the normal bright parenchyma and the surrounding hypointense retroperitoneal fat [41]. Coronal and axial magnetic resonance cholangiopancreatography (MRCP) with SSFSE accurately depicts the pancreatic ducts.

For the evaluation of PanNENs, fat-suppressed three-dimensional spoiled GRE sequences after the administration of gadolinium-DTPA are acquired in arterial phase (30–40 s), portal phase (70–80 s), and equilibrium phase (180 s) [13, 40, 41]. The acquired images should cover the upper abdomen, including the entire liver, thus improving the detection and characterization of loco-regional lymph-nodes and hepatic lesions [13].

Similar to contrast-enhanced helical CT, additional gadolinium enhanced scans can be obtained in the early arterial (scan delay 20 s) or late venous (120 s) phases, which increases the possibility of imaging the typical hypervascular enhancement pattern of these tumors [13, 31, 42].

9.4.2 Imaging Findings

On T1-weighted images, the normal pancreas exhibits medium to high signal intensity, similar to or slightly less than that of liver, but lower than that of retroperitoneal fat.

Fat suppression should be used, especially for T1 sequences, to increase pancreatic conspicuity, since with this technique the pancreas assumes a bright signal intensity that facilitates the detection of focal lesions [41, 42]. In patients with fatty involution of the pancreas, the signal intensity of this organ increases on T1-weighted sequences according to the amount of fat present within the parenchyma. Consequently, the pancreatic bed appears as an area of very low signal intensity on fat-sat sequences, which therefore are of little use in the visualization of small tumors (Fig. 9.12).

T2-weighted images with fat suppression may be useful for the evaluation of peri-pancreatic structures and inflammatory changes, but they are not strictly needed for imaging panNENs. On TSE T2-weighted images, the pancreas

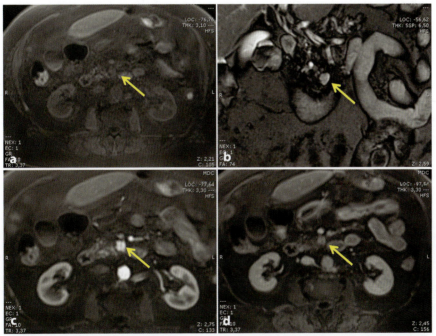

Fig. 9.12 Typical MRI finings of insulinoma. The on baseline unenhanced scan shows the lesion (*arrow*) as hypointense on the fat-saturated, T1-weighted, axial image (**a**) and hyperintense on the coronal T2-weighted image (**b**). During the contrast-enhanced study, the lesion (*arrow*) shows the typical hypervascularity on axial images obtained during the arterial pancreatic phase (**c**) and subsequent washout during late venous phase (**d**)

demonstrates intermediate signal intensity, similar to that of the liver. The signal may be intermediate to low on HASTE sequences.

The surface of the normal pancreatic parenchyma may be either smooth or lobulated.

Pancreatic ducts appear as low-signal intensity tubular structures on T1-weighted sequences and as high-signal intensity structures on heavily T2-weighted scans. At MRCP, heavy T2-weighting and fat suppression provide a cholangiogram useful for the evaluation of pancreatic and biliary duct involvement.

The typical MRI features of panNENs include a pancreatic mass of low signal intensity on T1-weighted images and of intermediate to high intensity on T2-weighted images (Fig. 9.12). As previously stated, the better intrinsic contrast resolution of this imaging technique may be advantageous for the identification of very small primary tumors, which frequently appear hypointense relative to the normal parenchyma on T1-weighted sequences. Lesion conspicuity is usually enhanced by fat-suppression.

Small lesions, which account for the majority of F-panNENs and some incidentally detected NF-PanNENs, are often quite homogeneous. Conversely, larger tumors may appear markedly inhomogeneous due to intralesional necrosis or hemorrhage, which may be seen as hyperintensity on T1-weighted images [43] and inhomogeneous hyperintensity on T2-weighted images (Fig. 9.13).

Cystic tumors have been described [35] and are often associated with widespread intralesional necrosis. Cystic lesions are usually unilocular, with contents that are hypointense on T1-weighted and hyperintense on T2-weighted images [44]. The cystic wall may show variable thickness [44]. The appearance of these tumors may be similar or even identical to that of other cystic tumors of the pancreas. Sometimes, intense enhancement of a peripheral ring-shaped viable tumor will suggest the diagnosis of cystic NF-panNENs (Fig. 9.14); however, in the majority of cases, a definitive diagnosis can only be obtained by histological examination of the resected specimen.

Among their atypical features, some islet tumors may have a low signal intensity on T2-weighted images due to the presence of abundant fibrous tissue [45]; in such cases they may be indistinguishable from ductal adenocarcinoma.

As seen for CT, during dynamic contrast-enhanced study, the majority of PanNENs show a typical hypervascularity [13, 31, 33, 46], resulting in hyperintense lesions compared to normal pancreatic and liver parenchyma (Figs. 9.11c, d, 9.12, 9.13).

In general, small tumors are depicted as homogeneously enhancing lesions (Fig. 9.12), whereas large tumors may appear markedly inhomogeneous during dynamic studies, since central necrotic areas remain hypointense on T1-weighted images even after contrast medium administration (Fig. 9.13).

The highest signal intensity is most frequently reached in the pancreatic phase [13] although the lesions may remain hyperintense during the portal

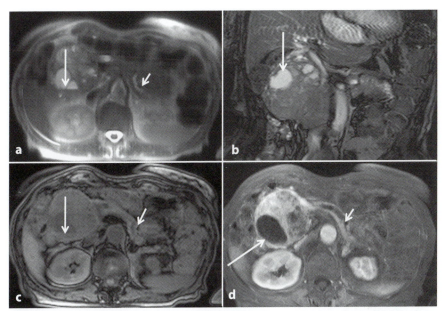

Fig. 9.13 Typical MRI findings of large NF-PanNEN/Cs. Pre-contrast examination shows a large tumor of the pancreatic head with upstream dilatation of the main pancreatic duct (*short arrow*). The lesion is markedly inhomogeneous on axial (**a**) and coronal (**b**) T2-weighted images and on the axial T1-weighted image, presenting intralesional necrosis and cystic changes with a fluid-fluid level (*long arrow*). After gadolinium administration (**d**), tumor inhomogeneity due to cystic change is confirmed (*long arrow*)

enhanced phase [30, 45]. Alternatively, some lesions may show early washout during the portal and late venous phases.

Persistent hyperintensity during late enhanced phases is found mainly in the larger lesions, where the neoplastic thrombosis of the draining veins results in retention of contrast medium [30].

The usefulness of delayed gadolinium-enhanced T1-weighted images (obtained 5–10 min following injection) has been postulated in scirrous tumors, showing delayed enhancement [31] (Fig. 9.15).

As for CT, the best dynamic phase for studying endocrine tumors is still a matter of debate; however, without any radiation exposure, modern fast breath-hold sequences should be used to obtain multiple contrast-enhanced phases during dynamic study, including early arterial, arterial pancreatic, portal venous, and late venous phases.

Multi-phasic dynamic study enhances the likelihood of detecting liver metastases, frequently imaged as hypervascular hepatic lesions [13, 36, 45] during the arterial pancreatic phase (Fig. 9.16). Metastases can also be depicted as hypovascular focal liver lesions during portal and late venous phases.

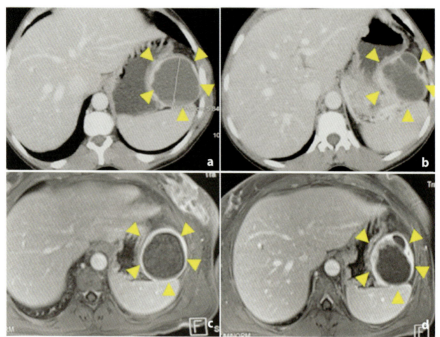

Fig. 9.14 Cystic PanNEN studied using MDCT and MRI. A large cystic PanNEN of the pancreatic tail can be recognized on the axial images acquired during portal venous phase, both at MDCT (**a, b**) and at MRI (**c, d**). The ring-shaped pattern of enhancement (*arrowheads*) is better depicted on the latter. A differential diagnosis with other cystic pancreatic tumors cannot be obtained in this case

The value of liver-specific Gd-chelates in the identification of both primary pancreatic tumor and hepatic metastases has been reported [47, 48]. Delayed hepato-biliary phase, obtained after the administration of liver-specific contrast material, can detect small metastases that other sequences may have failed to demonstrate [48].

9.5   Other Radiologic Diagnostic Tests

Before non-invasive cross-sectional imaging methods were introduced, selective arteriography of the proper or common hepatic artery, the gastroduodenal, splenic, superior mesenteric, and at times the dorsal pancreatic artery was the principal technique for localizing these hypervascular endocrine tumors of the pancreas. The arteriographic appearance of all islet cell tumors is similar for F-PanNENs and NF-PanNENs. It is not possible to distinguish a functioning from a non-functioning tumor or one type of functioning tumor from another. However, the marked hypervascularity and intense homogeneous staining permit

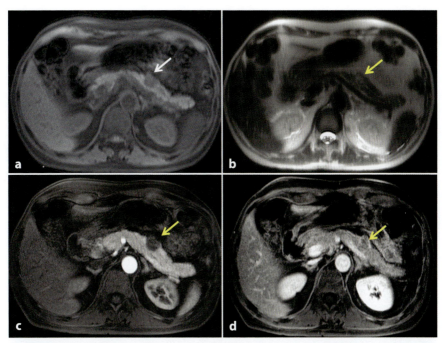

Fig. 9.15 Atypical delayed enhancement of a PanNEN of the pancreatic body. A relatively small NF-PanNEN is hypointense on the pre-contrast T1-weighted image (**a**) and slightly hyperintense on the T2-weighted image (**b**). The tumor is hypovascularized during the arterial pancreatic phase (**c**) but shows delayed enhancement, resulting in an isointense lesion with a thin hyperintense rim on the enhanced axial image acquired at the time of late venous phase (**d**)

the distinction of PanNENs from other tumors such as pancreatic adenocarcinoma [49]. Arterial and venous involvement can often be demonstrated in larger lesions.

Neovascularity and portal vein invasion indicate that the tumor is malignant.

Portal venous sampling (PVS), also called pancreatic venous sampling or trans-hepatic venous sampling, involves catheterization of the portal vein using a trans-hepatic approach [50]. The branches of the extrahepatic portal venous system are selectively catheterized and blood samples obtained. The sample with the highest concentration of tumor cells comes from the vein that drains the area of the tumor.

In case of arterial stimulation with venous sampling, the tumor is stimulated to secrete hormones by a specific injected secretagogue, and venous samples are obtained from the right and left hepatic veins [49] at 0.5, 1, and 2 min after each injection. If the hormone concentration increases, the arterial supply to the tumor can be identified and therefore the region where the tumor is located. If the hormone concentration increases after the drug has

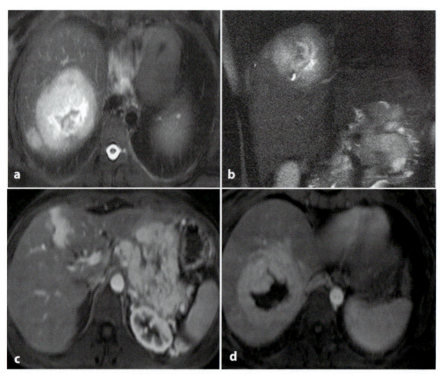

Fig. 9.16 Liver metastases studied using MRI. Large metastases appear homogeneously hyperintense on the T2-weighted image (**a, b**). Small metastases are hypervascular during arterial pancreatic phase (**c**), whereas a large lesion may show inhomogeneity due to central necrosis (**d**)

been injected into the proper hepatic artery, the presence of hepatic metastases can be diagnosed.

Based on the measurement of the hormone concentration in each venous sample, these diagnostic methods were employed in the past for evaluating functioning tumors. However, due to high cost and relative invasiveness, these tools are no longer used in clinical routine.

9.6 Imaging Features of Functioning F-PanNENs

Among the islet cell tumors of the pancreas, insulinoma is the most common endocrine tumor, followed by gastrinoma, VIPoma, glucagonoma, somatostatinoma, and other, rarely encountered pancreatic secretory tumors.

In functioning tumors, the clinical data and laboratory tests often permit an accurate clinical diagnosis, so that cross-sectional imaging is used to localize the tumor within or eventually outside the pancreas, guiding the surgeon to the appropriate tumor resection.

9 Imaging

Patients suffering from MEN1 pose a radiologic challenge, because of the possibility of multiple pancreatic and extrapancreatic tumors (mainly located in the duodenal or gastric wall).

9.6.1 Insulinoma

Insulinomas are frequently small at detection, often measuring < 2 cm, at diagnosis due to the fact that symptoms related to hypoglycemia can occur even with small amounts of insulin.

Most insulinomas (90%) are benign solitary lesions; sporadic lesions are more frequently encountered in women (60%), especially between the fifth and sixth decades of life.

Malignancy should be suspected in case of large (> 2 cm) lesions or intralesional calcifications.

The appearance of liver metastases is similar to that of the primary tumor, i.e., hypervascular during arterial phases and showing washout during portal and late venous phases.

Patients suffering from MEN1 tend to present with multiple tumors, especially in case of presentation at a young age.

On abdominal US, when detectable according to their location and to patient habitus, insulinomas may appear as hypoechoic lesions compared to normal parenchyma; however, in many cases they are iso-echocic with respect to the surrounding parenchyma. In addition, due to their frequently small size, a mass effect cannot be considered as a reliable finding for lesion detection. When a tumor is visualized or suspected on the basis of a baseline scan, the intravenous administration of sonographic contrast material may help in its identification, as it typically appears at CEUS as a hypervascular focal lesion [17].

Endoscopic ultrasound provides excellent results for tumors in the head of the pancreas (sensitivity 83%) but poor sensitivity (38%) for those located in the tail [21].

On CT, these lesions are usually isodense to normal parenchyma on baseline scan. The presence of calcifications may help in the detection of a small lesion, especially in case of poorly enhancing lesions.

The majority of insulinomas appear as brightly enhancing, round to oval masses that demonstrate rapid washout in the portal and late venous phases [33]. Over two-thirds are located to the left of the superior mesenteric artery [51].

Iso-vascular or hypovascular lesions are difficult to localize and may require additional imaging studies for lesion identification.

On MRI, insulinomas frequently show low signal intensity on T1-weighted fat-suppressed images and high signal intensity on T2-weighted images [52]. However, some tumors may be iso-intense to the pancreas on pre-contrast T1 sequences. Occasionally, an insulinoma can show low signal intensity on T2-weighted sequences due to the presence of a fibrous or sclero-hyaline stroma [52]. Diffusion-weighted sequences and the ADC map may help in the identification of these tumors based on their high sensitivity and contrast resolution [42].

Most insulinomas show intense enhancement with gadolinium throughout the lesion, and some may demonstrate ring-like peripheral enhancement [53]. The presence of fibrous tissue diminishes the degree of enhancement during the early dynamic study and may be associated with delayed enhancement in some instances.

In conclusion, MDCT and MRI are the best imaging techniques for preoperatively diagnosing small pancreatic insulinomas, but in either case optimal technique and state-of-the-art equipment are mandatory. In cases in which CT, MRI, EUS, and scintigraphy results are negative, IOUS at the time of surgical resection represents the last opportunity to confirm these tumors in patients in whom strong clinical suspicion persists, and/or to find additional tumors. IOUS is particularly important in patients with multiple lesions and MEN1 since under these conditions ectopic tumors, which may be multiple, are quite frequent and difficult to find with CT or MRI [27].

9.6.2 Gastrinoma

Gastrinomas are usually larger than insulinomas at diagnosis (> 2 cm), multiple in 60% of patients, malignant in 60–65%, and associated with MEN1 in 20–60%.

Most of these tumors are located in the so-called gastrinoma triangle (between the junction of the head and neck of the pancreas, the second and third portion of the duodenum, the junction of the cystic duct and the common bile duct). Although gastrinomas are usually slow growing, approximately 50% of patients with gastrinoma have metastases at the time of diagnosis.

Gastrinomas are hypervascular tumors. They are best visualized by using thin-slice sections and a dual-phase CT protocol, with arterial and portal venous phases [54, 55]. The imaging technique is therefore similar to that used for other functioning tumors.

Due to their larger size, pancreatic gastrinomas are usually easily detected by MDCT; however, ectopically located tumors are more challenging.

Metastases to the liver and loco-regional lymph-nodes tend to be similar in appearance to the primary tumor [36].

MRI can also be employed for the identification and staging of gastrinomas, with some studies reporting sensitivities of 20–62% [54, 55].

EUS was shown to be cost-effective compared with a control group examined by venous sampling [56].

Results with angiography vary greatly across studies [54]. CT and MRI have the advantage of staging the entire abdomen and pelvis, which is not possible with the limited depth penetration of EUS. In equivocal or negative cases with a high clinical suspicion, somatostatin-receptor scintigraphy is very effective in assessing both the primary tumor in the pancreas or ectopic sites and metastatic lesions to the liver.

9.6.3 VIPoma

On average, these tumors share similar imaging feature with other functioning endocrine tumors. VIPomas are usually > 3 cm in diameter at the time of diagnosis and may be malignant in over 60% of the cases [57, 58].

The majority of the neoplasms are located in the body or tail of the pancreas [58]. Occasionally, tumors causing a similar clinical syndrome are located in the adrenal glands, retroperitoneum, ganglia of sympathetic chain, lung, and as intestinal carcinoids [57, 58]. Rarely, these tumors are associated with MEN1 [59]. Statistical data concerning the accuracy of imaging studies are not available.

MDCT, MRI, US, and angiography have been used to localize the primary lesion and to identify metastases. On contrast-enhanced imaging studies, the latter, mainly involving the liver, frequently show intense enhancement similar to the appearance of the primary tumor.

9.6.4 Glucagonoma

Glucagonomas are intrapancreatic tumors mostly involving the head and neck of the gland.

They occur with a slight prevalence in women, with a peak age of 55 years [60]. The tumor is malignant in about 60% of patients, and the 5-year survival is 50%. When not diagnosed on the basis of clinical and laboratory findings, glucagonomas become symptomatic, causing symptoms related to mass effect, locoregional infiltration, and lymph node and liver metastases.

CT, MR, angiography, and US have been used successfully to diagnose and stage these tumors, but in all reports the conclusions were based only on anecdotal references [10, 61].

9.6.5 Somatostatinoma

Somatostatinomas are usually solitary, aggressive lesions occurring in the fourth to sixth decades of life. Metastases at the time of diagnosis have been described in more than 70% of patients in some series [62]. This tumor is usually located within the pancreas, where it tends to be quite large (2–10 cm in diameter); 75% occur in the head [51].

However, somatostatinomas may also arise within small bowel loops, the duodenal ampulla, or the peri-ampullary region [62].

A prevalence of duodenal locations for men and pancreatic locations for women has been described [63]. When the small bowel is involved, the neoplasm can be considered as a carcinoid that consists almost completely of somatostatin-containing cells but produces little somatostatin.

Extrapancreatic lesions, with a mean diameter of about 2 cm, are frequently diagnosed early because of the presence of symptoms such as jaundice, bleeding, and ulcerations.

The radiologic features of somatostatinomas resemble those of other neuroendocrine tumors.

Imaging studies usually demonstrate a hypervascular lesion, with or without hypervascular lymph nodes and liver metastases [64].

The demonstration of ectopically located tumors, involving the duodenum or intestinal loop, may be challenging for radiologists. In suspected cases, a dedicated protocol including filling of the duodenal and intestinal loops with water or oral contrast material may facilitate the detection of ectopically located primary tumors.

9.6.7 Other F-PanNENs

Other, very rare functioning endocrine tumors of the pancreas have been occasionally described, including corticotropinoma, ACTHoma, and GRFoma. Their clinical diagnosis is challenging because they are clinically not associated with a specific endocrine syndrome.

Like all the other functioning endocrine tumors, these rare neoplasms usually demonstrate the features of a hypervascular mass without or with liver metastases.

9.7 Diagnostic Strategies for F-PanNENs

Functioning endocrine tumors of the pancreas continue to challenge the radiologist. Earlier reports showed that up to 27% of patients have tumors not detected preoperatively with either helical CT or MRI. Sensitivities that approach 90–95% for lesions located in the pancreatic head region are achieved with EUS, but its sensitivity is limited for lesions located in the tail; also, EUS cannot be used for reliable preoperative staging.

Ectopically located, extra-pancreatic F-NENs are likewise imaged with difficulty, especially when they are small in diameter.

Overall, arteriography and venous sampling are no longer routinely employed even in difficult cases, because of the inherent technical problems associated with the test and the higher cost.

More recently, somatostatin-receptor scintigraphy and positron emission tomography have been used to establish or confirm the presence of ectopic lesions or small masses suspected on CT or MRI, and to improve results in assessing metastatic disease.

The best results are reportedly obtained with a combination of intraoperative palpation and IOUS due to their complementary nature during surgery.

Somatostatin-receptor techniques can be used for treatment and to monitor its success in patients with functioning tumors of the pancreas [65].

9.8 Diagnostic Strategies for NF-PanNENs

In most cases, NF-PanNENs are found by chance in patients suffering from non-specific symptoms (palpable mass, dyspepsia, etc.). In these settings, the diagnosis is usually late, and either US or CT is the first method to suggest the diagnosis. With the recent increase in the number and quality of cross-sectional imaging studies, a significant percentage of these lesions are discovered incidentally in asymptomatic patients.

The role of the radiologist is to characterize the lesion, demonstrating the typical hypervascular enhancement pattern, using CT, MRI, or CEUS.

However, since a definite characterization is not objectively possible with imaging, fine-needle biopsy is always advisable before treatment.

The prognosis of patients with NF-PanNENs is much better than that of patients with ductal adenocarcinomas, and therefore a surgical attempt integrated with chemotherapy is indicated even in more advanced stages of the disease. Accurate staging of the tumor can be obtained with CT or MRI [13].

MDCT and MRI findings are virtually identical: but based on its wide availability and slightly higher accuracy in preoperative staging, the former should be considered as the imaging tool of choice [13].

Nuclear medicine could improve tumor staging, as it is able to identify distant metastases and to assess the potential benefits of treatment with somatostatin analogues, either cold or radiolabeled. The presence of somatostatin receptor subtype 2 is promising in terms of treatment success. Moreover, in the follow-up of these tumors, due to the further advantage of identifying distant metastases, nuclear medicine techniques may be advisable, given that CT and MRI are able to distinguish scar tissue from the residual or relapsing tumor only with difficulty, especially in operated patients.

9.9 Differential Diagnosis

The diagnosis of F-PanNENs usually does not pose any dilemmas. Problems that arise in the differential diagnosis between NF-PanNENs and the other pancreatic masses vary according to the radiological aspect of the tumor, which in turn is strictly dependent on its vascular behavior.

The most typical variant of NF-PanNENs, characterized by a solid hypervascularized appearance at imaging, is usually easily diagnosed on CT, MRI, and CEUS due to its conspicuous enhancement after contrast medium administration. Characterization of these tumors is also facilitated by the presence of hypervascularized hepatic metastases.

Rare tumors that show a hypervascular enhancement pattern during the arterial pancreatic phase and potentially mimicking the solid variant of NF-PanNENs include acinar carcinoma [66] and serous cystadenoma, in their solid variant [67]. Ductal adenocarcinoma, in rare cases, exhibits strong enhancement, necessitating a differential diagnosis.

Finally, hypervascularized pancreatic metastases, especially from renal tumors, must be taken into account, since they may have the same pattern [68]. However, the differential diagnosis is simple if there is a known primary tumor and other synchronous or metachronous metastases.

Moreover, pancreatic metastases, which can appear many years after identification of the primary tumor, are frequently multiple.

The solid hypovascularized variant of NF-PanNEN cannot be reliably characterized using cross-sectional imaging, and biopsy is always needed. If an infiltrating growth pattern is depicted at imaging, with or without associated hypovascularized liver metastases, imaging will not allow the differential diagnosis with pancreatic adenocarcinoma.

When the tumor presents as an expansive growth pattern with well-defined contours, especially in young women, the differential diagnosis must include a solid pseudopapillary tumor.

Finally, rare cystic endocrine tumors cannot be differentiated on the basis of imaging findings from mucinous cystic tumors (especially unilocular lesions) or solid pseudopapillary tumors in their cystic variant.

An intrapancreatic accessory spleen should be considered in the differential diagnosis of F-NENs and NF-PanNENs. It can be ruled out based on differences in vascular behavior, or in some cases in signal intensity at baseline MRI.

References

1. Kaltsas GA, Besser GM, Grossman AB (2004) The diagnosis and medical management of advanced neuroendocrine tumors. Endocr Rev 25:458-511
2. Eriksson B, Oberg K (2000) Neuroendocrine tumours of the pancreas. Br J Surg 87:129-131
3. Lam KY, Lo CY (1997) Pancreatic endocrine tumour: a 22-year clinicopathological experience with morphological, immunohistochemical observation and a review of the literature. Eur J Surg Oncol 23:36-42
4. Hoff A, Cote G, Gagel R (2004) Management of neuroendocrine cancers of the gastrointestinal tract: islet cell carcinoma of the pancreas and other neuroendocrine carcinomas. In: Abbruzzese J, Evans D, Willett C, Fenoglio-Preiser C (eds.) Gastrointestinal oncology. Oxford University Press, New York, pp. 780-800
5. Solcia E, Capella C, Kloppel G (1997) Tumors of the pancreas, vol fasc 20. AFIP atlas of tumor pathology, 3rd edn. Armed Forces Institute of Pathology, Washington DC
6. Dixon E, Pasieka JL (2007) Funtioning and nonfuntioning neuroendocrine tumors of the pancreas. Curr Opin Oncol 19:30-35

7. Rockall AG, Reznek RH (2007) Imaging of neuroendocrine tumours (CT/RM/US). Best Pract Res Clin Endocrinol Metab 21:43-68
8. Modlin IM, Oberg K, Chung DC et al (2008) Gastroenteropancreatic neuroendocrine tumours. Lancet Oncol 9:61-72
9. Kloppel G, Heitz PU (1988) Pancreatic endocrine tumors. Pathol Res Pract 183:155-168
10. Phan GQ, Yeo CJ, Hruban RH et al (1998) Surgical experience with pancreatic and peripancreatic neuroendocrine tumors: review of 125 patients. J Gastrointest Surg 2:472-482
11. Falconi M, Bonora A, Bassi C et al (2000). In: Pederzoli P, Bassi C (eds) Pancreatic tumors. Achievement and prospective. Thieme, Struttugart, pp. 368-397
12. Falconi M, Bettini R, Boninsegna L et al (2006) Surgical strategy in the treatment of pancreatic neuroendocrine tumors. JOP 7:150-156
13. Foti G, Boninsegna L, Falconi M, Pozzi Mucelli R (2012) Preoperative assessment of nonfunctioning pancreatic endocrine tumors: role of MDCT and MRI. Rad Med (in press)
14. Solcia E, Kloppel G, Sobin L et al (2000) Histological typing of endocrine tumours. World Health Organization International Histological Classification of Tumours, 2nd edn. Springer, Berlin
15. Fugazzola C, Procacci C, Bergamo Andreis IA et al (1990) The contribution of ultrasonography and computed tomography in the diagnosis of nonfunctioning islet cell tumors of the pancreas. Gastrointest Radiol 15:139-44
16. Hessel SI, Siegelman SS, McNeil BI (1982) A prospective evaluation of computed tomography and ultrasound of the pancreas. Radiology 143:129-133
17. D'Onofrio M, Mansueto G, Vasori S (2003) Contrast enhanced ultrasonographic detection of small pancreatic insulinoma. J Ultrasound Med 22:4413-4417
18. D'Onofrio M, Zamboni G, Faccioli N et al (2007) Ultrasonography of the pancreas. Contrast-enhanced imaging. Abdominal Imaging 32:171-181
19. D'Onofrio M, Malagò R, Zamboni G et al (2005) Contrast-enhanced ultrasonography better identifies pancreatic tumor vascolarization than helical CT. Pancreatology 5:398-402
20. D'Onofrio M, Mansueto G, Falconi M et al (2004) Neuroendocrine pancreatic tumor: value of contrast enhanced ultrasonography. Abdom Imaging 29:246-258
21. Schumacher B, Liibke HI, Frieling T (1996) Prospective study on the detection of insulinomas by endoscopic ultrasonography. Endoscopy 28:273-276
22. Gress FG, Barawi M, Kim D, Grendell IH (2002) Preoperative localization of a neuroendocrine tumor of the pancreas with EUS-guided line needle tattooing. Gastrointest Endosc 55:594-597
23. Alsohaibani F, Bigam D, Kneteman N et al (2008) The impact of preoperative endoscopic ultrasound on the surgical management of pancreatic neuroendocrine tumours. Can J Gastroenterol 22:817-820
24. Gunther RW, Klose KI, Ruckert K et al (1985) Localization of small islet-cell tumors. Preoperative and intraoperative ultrasound, computed tomography, arteriography digital subtraction angiography, and pan-creatic venous sampling. Gastrointest Radiol 10:145-152
25. Malagò R, D'Onofrio M, Zamboni GA et al (2009). Contrast-enhanced sonography of nonfunctioning pancreatic neuroendocrine tumors. Am J Roentgenol 192:424-30
26. Hayakawa T, Iin CX, Hirooka Y (2000) Endoscopic ultrasonography of the pancreas: new advances. IOP 1:46-48
27. Lewis MA, Thompson GB, Young WF Jr (2012) Preoperative Assessment of the Pancreas in Multiple Endocrine Neoplasia Type 1. World J Surg [Epub ahead of print]
28. Procacci C, Carbognin G, Accordini S et al (2001) Nonfunctioning endocrine tumors of the pancreas: possibilities of spiral CT characterization. Eur Radiol 11:1175-1183
29. Iglesias A, Arias M, Casal M et al (2001) Unusual presentation of a pancreatic insulinoma in helical CT and dynamic contrast-enhanced MR imaging: case report. Eur Radiol 11:926-930
30. Stafford Iohnson DB, Francis IR, Eckhauser FE et al (1998) Dual-phase helical CT of nonfunctioning islet cell tumors. Comput Assist Tomogr 22:59-63
31. Ichikawa T, Peterson MS, Federle MP et al (2000) lslet cell tumor of the pancreas: biphasic CT versus MR imaging in tumor detection. Radiology 216:163-171

32. McNulty NI, Francis 1R, Platt IF et al (2001) Multi-detector row helical CT of is pancreas: effect of contrast-enhanced multiphasic imaging on enhancement of the pancreas, peripancreatic vasculature and pancreatic adenocarcinoma. Radiology 220:97-102
33. Graziani R, Brandalise A, Bellotti M et al (2010). Imaging of neuroendocrine gastroenteropancreatic tumours. Radiol Med 115:1047-1064
34. Chung MI, Choi BI, Han IK et al (1997) Functioning islet cell tumor of the pancreas. Localization with dynamic spiral CT. Acta Radiol 38:135-138
35. Boninsegna L, Partelli S, D'Innocenzio MM et al (2010) Pancreatic cystic endocrine tumors: a different morphological entity associated with a less aggressive behavior. Neuroendocrinology 92:246-251
36. Debray MP, Geoffroy O, Laissy IP et al (2001) Imaging appearances of metastases from neuroendocrine tumours of the pancreas. Br I Radiol 74:1065-1070
37. Keogan MT, McDermott VG, Paulson EK et al (1997) Pancreatic malignancy: effect of dualphase helical CT in tumor detection and vascular opacification. Radiology 205:513-518
38. Van Hoe L, Gryspeerdt S, Marchal G et al (1995) Helical CT for the preoperative localization of islet cell tumors of the pancreas: value of arterial and parenchymal phase images. Am J Roentgenol 165:1437-1439
39. Koito K, Namieno T, Nagakawa T, Morita K (1997) Delayed enhancement of islet cell carcinoma on dynamic computed tomography: a sign of its malignancy. Abdom Imaging 22:304-306
40. Kalra MK, Maher MM, Mueller PR et al (2003) State-of-the-art imaging of pancreatic neoplasms. Br J Radiol76:857-865
41. Sung ER, Seung EJ, Kang HL et al (2007) CT and MR imaging findings of endocrine tumor of the pancreas according to WHO classification. European Journal of Radiology 62 371–377
42. Caramella C, Dromain C, De Baere T et al (2010) Endocrine pancreatic tumours: which are the most useful MRI sequences? Eur Radiol 20:2618-27
43. Carlson B, Iohnson CD, Stephens DH et al (1993) MRI of pancreatic islet cell carcinoma. J Comput Assist Tomogr 17:735-740
44. Buetow PC, Miller DL, Parrino TV, Buck IL (1997) lslet cell tumors of the pancreas: clinical, radiologic, and pathologic correlation in diagnosis and localization. Radiographics 17:453-472
45. Owen NI, Sohaib SA, Peppercorn PD et al (2001) MRI of pancreatic neuroendocrine tumours. Br I Radiol 74:968-973
46. Lewis RB, Lattin GE, Paal E (2010). Pancreatic endocrine tumors: radiologicalclinicopathological correlation. Radiographics 30:1445-64
47. Petersein I, Spinazzi A, Giovagnoni A et al (2000) Focal liver lesions: evaluation of the eficacy of gadobenate dimeglumine in MR imaging - a multicenter phase III clinical study. Radiology 215:727-736
48. Motosugi U, Ichikawa T, Morisaka H et al (2011) Detection of Pancreatic Carcinoma and Liver Metastases with Gadoxetic Acid-enhanced MR Imaging: Comparison with contrast-enhanced multi-detector row CT. Radiology 260:446-453
49. Doppman IL, Nieman L, Miller DL et al (1989) Ectopic adrenocorticotropic hormone syndrome: localization studies in 28 patients. Radiology 172:115-124
50. Vinik A1, Moattari AR, Cho K, Thompson N (1990) Transhepatic portal vein catheterization for localization of sporadic and MEN gastrinomas: a ten-year experience. Surgery 107:246-255
51. Howard TI, Stabile BE, Zinner MI et al (1990) Anatomic distribution of pancreatic endocrine tumors. Am I Surg 159:258-264
52. Thoeni RF, Mueller-Lisse UG, Chan R et al (2001) Detection of small, functional islet cell tumors in the pancreas: selection of MRI Imaging sequences for optimal sensitivity. Radiology 214:483-490
53. Kraus BB, Ros PR (1994) Insulinoma: diagnosis with fat-suppressed MR imaging. AJR 162:69-70
54. Frucht H, Doppman IL, Norton IA et al (1989) Gastrinomas: comparison of MR imaging with CT, angiography, and US. Radiology 171:713-717

55. Pisegna IR, Doppman IL, Norton IA et al (1993) Prospective comparative study of the ability of MR imaging and other imaging modalities to localize tumors in patients with Zollinger-Ellison syndrome. Dig Dis Sci 38:1318-1328
56. Bansal R, Tierney W, Carpenter S et al (1999) Cost effectiveness of EUS for preoperative localization of pancreatic endocrine tumors. Gastrointest Endosc 49:19-25
57. Kloppel G, Heitz PU (1988) Pancreatic endocrine tumors Pathol Res Pract 183:155-168
58. Iaffe BM (1987) Surgery for gut hormone-producing tumors. Am I Med 82:68-76
59. Krejs GI (1987) V1Poma syndrome. Am I Med 82:37-48
60. Bloom SR, Polak IM (1987) Glucagonoma syndrome. Am J Med 82:25-36
61. Solivetti FM, Giunta S, Caterino M et al (2001) CT findings in a case of glucagonoma with necrolytic migrating erythema. Radiol Med (Torino) 102:410-412
62. Tanaka S, Yamasaki S, Matsushita H et al (2000) Duodenal somatostatinoma: a case report and review of 31 cases with special reference to the relationship between tumor size and metastasis. Pathol Int 50:146-152
63. Patel YC, Ganda OP, Benoit R (1983) Pancreatic somatostatinoma: abundance of somatostatin-28(1-12)-like immunoreactivity in tumor and plasma. I Clin Endocrinol Metab 57:1048-1053
64. Semelka RC, Custodio CM, Cem Balci N, Woosley IT (2000) Neuroendocrine tumors of the pancreas: spectrum of appearances on MRI. I Magn Reson Imaging 11:141-148
65. Ugur O, Kothari PI, Finn RD et al (2002) Ga-66 labeled somatostatin analogue DOTA-DPhe1-Tyr3-octreotide as a potential agent for positron emission tomography imaging and receptor mediated internal radiotherapy of somatostatin receptor positive tumors. Nucl Med Biol 29:147-157
66. Ogawa T, Isaji S, Yabana T (2000) A case of mixed acinar endocrine carcinoma of the pancreas discovered in an asymptomatic subject. Int I Pancreatol 27:249-257
67. Gabata T, Terayama N, Yamashiro M et al (2005) Solid serous cystadenoma of the pancreas: MR imaging with pathologic correlation. Abdom Imaging 30:605-609
68. Ghavamian R, Klein KA, Stephens DH et al (2000) Renal cell carcinoma metastatic to the pancreas: clinical and radiological features. Mayo Clin Proc 75:581-585

Surgical Therapy

10

Rossella Bettini, Stefano Partelli, Stefano Crippa,
Letizia Boninsegna and Massimo Falconi

10.1 Introduction

The surgical management of pancreatic neuroendocrine neoplasm (PanNEN) is often challenging due to the heterogeneous presentation and the different biological behavior of these neoplasms. Recent research advances have led to more accurate recommendations for the management of these tumors [1-3]. This chapter summarizes the state of the art concerning the indications for surgery and the optimal surgical approach of sporadic tumors as well as PanNENs associated with multiple endocrine neoplasm type 1 (MEN1) syndrome.

10.2 Sporadic Disease

Surgery of sporadic PanNENs should be tailored according to the stage of the disease and the biological behavior of the tumor(s).

10.2.1 Functioning PanNENs of Unknown Primary

When primary tumor cannot be assessed but the presence of a hormonal syndrome related to endocrine pancreatic tumor hypersecretion has been ascertained, the main aim is to identify the lesion. Despite the widespread use of high-quality imaging techniques, insulinomas and gastrinomas remain undetected in 10-20% of cases [4, 5]. However, the absence of a preoperative local-

---

M. Falconi (✉)
Department of Surgery and Oncology, "G.B. Rossi" University Hospital, Verona, Italy
and General Surgery Unit, "Sacro Cuore – Don Calabria" Hospital,
Negrar (VR), Italy
e-mail: massimo.falconi@univr.it

P. Pederzoli and C. Bassi (eds.), *Uncommon Pancreatic Neoplasms*,
Updates in Surgery
DOI: 10.1007/978-88-470-2673-5_10, © Springer-Verlag Italia 2013

109

ization should not be considered a contraindication for surgery in patients with proven functional disease.

In these cases, an exploratory laparotomy should include a careful abdominal inspection of the liver, stomach, and mesentery. The pancreatic gland should be well exposed according to the Kocher maneuver and its superior and inferior margins accurately dissected. The entire pancreatic gland is then accessible for a bi-digital manual examination and the parenchyma can be thoroughly explored by intraoperative ultrasound (IOUS) with a 7.5- or 10-MHz probe. Macroscopically, insulinomas appear as gray-reddish masses, with a harder consistency than the surrounding parenchyma; the ultrasound examination reveals a hypoechogeneic aspect. An intraoperative localization, as determined by IOUS, can be achieved in 92–98% of the cases [4-6]. IOUS can also assess the relationship of the tumor with the main pancreatic duct, guiding the surgeon in an enucleation or a standard pancreatic resection.

Whereas IOUS is able to identify nearly 91% of pancreatic gastrinomas, the detection rate decreases to approximately 30% for duodenal gastrinomas. In this setting, pancreatic exploration must be followed by a trans-illumination of the duodenum and a 3-cm incision of the descending duodenum, in order to assess the medial wall, where the majority of gastrinomas are found. The accuracy of duodenotomy is indeed higher than either palpation alone or IOUS imaging associated with trans-illumination [4, 5]. The surgical procedure should also include a resection of the peri-pancreatic lymph nodes as well as a lymphadenectomy of the celiac trunk and hepatic ligament, based on the risk of a primary lymph node gastrinoma.

In all cases, a careful intraoperative examination of the specimen by the pathologist is mandatory in order to confirm the presence of the lesion.

If this protocol fails, "blind" resections are discouraged and patients should undergo strict follow-up while the hypersecretion symptom is controlled by medical therapy [7].

10.2.2 Localized PanNENs

When a PanNEN is localized, surgery is the treatment of choice. Nevertheless with the advent of high-resolution imaging techniques, small non-functioning PanNENs are increasingly discovered, and it is now debated whether all small and asymptomatic lesions should be routinely resected [8]. In this subgroup of patients, non-operative management has been recently advocated for incidentally discovered PanNENs < 2 cm [9]. Although data on the non-operative management of these forms are still lacking, a strict yearly follow-up seems to be a reasonable recommendation. Any significant increasing in the size of these tumors should be promptly recognized and patients should be addressed to surgery.

The optimal surgical resection for localized PanNEN is still debated. Two main surgical approaches are currently available: typical (i.e., pancreaticoduodenectomy or left pancreatectomy with or without spleen preservation) and atypical (i.e., enucleation or middle pancreatectomy) resections. The surgical choice is based on technical considerations (site, proximity to Wirsung duct, etc.) and on the aggressiveness of the disease, which is mainly correlated with the size of the lesion [8, 9] and with the invasion of nearby organs. A typical pancreatic resection is always recommended in the presence of large PanNENs (main diameter > 2 cm), organ invasion and/or clinical symptoms. Typical pancreatic resections are associated with a high incidence of peri-operative complications as well as exocrine and endocrine insufficiency. These complications along with the increasingly incidental recognition of small and asymptomatic lesions have led to the increased use of parenchyma-sparing techniques or atypical resections, such as enucleation and middle pancreatectomy. Atypical resections have been proposed in the management of PanNENs, especially when they are well-demarcated and small in size [10]. In the absence of others signs of malignancies, tumor size represents the main criteria in the choice of the most appropriate surgical approach. Currently, a diameter of 2 cm seems to be reasonably safe for a limited resection [10]. A middle pancreatectomy can be appropriate for small tumors of the pancreatic body whereas an enucleation should be considered only if the main pancreatic duct can be safely preserved. Atypical resections reduce the risk of long-term endocrine/exocrine impairment as pancreatic parenchyma is spared by these techniques [11, 12]. However, atypical resections are associated with a high rate of pancreatic fistulas although the latter are mostly transient and with a low clinical impact [11]. Second-look surgery for those tumors with high-grade malignancy is mandatory after an atypical resection. Furthermore, the most recent guidelines suggest that nodal sampling with intraoperative pathological examination should be always performed [13].

10.2.3 Locally Advanced PanNENs

When a PanNEN is locally advanced and a potentially curative resection is feasible (R0–R1), a more aggressive surgical approach is justified. Several authors have demonstrated the benefit in terms of survival after pancreatic resection of locally advanced PanNENs when no residual macroscopic disease is present along the surgical margins [14].

Surgery always includes a typical pancreatic resection with standard lymphadenectomy, associated, if necessary, with nearby organ resection or vascular resection. Splenectomy is routinely performed in distal pancreatectomy. During this procedure, the adrenal gland, retroperitoneal tissue, and left kidney can be easily removed, if infiltrated. Tumors of the pancreatic head that involve the stomach can be removed by a Whipple procedure, while those infiltrating the colon require standard or segmental colon resection. When the entire pancreatic gland is involved, total pancreatectomy should be considered. A portal or superior mesenteric vein infiltration can occasionally occur;

in these cases, the surgeon can achieve negative resection margins by performing segmental resection of the superior mesenteric vein or splenomesenteric portal vein confluence. By contrast, an arterial resection is rarely performed when the mesenteric-celiac arterial axis is completely involved. The presence of celiac trunk invasion is not an absolute limitation for distal pancreatectomy, as prior reports have described efficacious dissection of the central-axis arteries or graft substitution; however, these procedures can be associated with severe diarrhea due to denervation of the intestinal plexa. The role of lymphadenectomy in these tumors is still a matter of debate, but a regional lymph node dissection along the hepatoduodenal ligament, celiac trunk, and superior mesenteric artery should be a standardized technique for invasive PanNENs.

When locally advanced pancreatic carcinomas present with massive local infiltration and resection would be incomplete, leaving macroscopic residual disease, there is no support for cytoreductive surgery (R2). A partial resection would, in fact, expose the patient to a high risk of bleeding and to the possible spread of tumor cells in the peritoneum. Recurrence, moreover, is the rule, with no guarantee of there being any advantage in terms of survival.

10.2.4 Metastatic PanNENs

Surgery also plays an important role in metastatic disease, although the presence of extra-abdominal disease should always be ruled out preoperatively. Hepatic surgery might require a wide range of different types of resections according to the number of liver metastases, their locations, and the hepatic reserve [15-17]. The operation can be performed as a one- or two-step procedure and always requires an accurate IOUS evaluation. Complete resection is associated with a 5-year survival rate of 60–80% compared with 30% in unresected patients [18-21]. However, due to the high incidence of multifocal and bilateral metastases, with liver involvement frequently exceeding 75%, a radical liver resection is possible in < 20% of patients [18]. However, recurrence is the rule, with a median time to progression of 16–20 months and a 5-year survival of 50–60% [22].

Debulking resections (R2) might be alternatively offered with palliative intent to all patients in whom 90% of the tumor burden can be safely removed, as part of a multimodal approach (combined or followed by other ablative therapy, peptide receptor radionuclide therapy, bio- and chemotherapy) [17]. Metastatic disease also can be treated by other interventional procedures [17, 23], mainly trans-arterial embolization (TAE), trans-arterial chemo-embolization (TACE), and radiofrequency ablation (RFA). Such procedures can be used as loco-regional ablative therapy per se or as an adjunct to palliative surgery. TAE or TACE are endovascular interventional radiology procedure that may be used to treat multiple or large liver metastases. Data regarding survival after TACE for metastatic PanNENs are still lacking although the procedure has been demonstrated as effective in reducing tumor size [24, 25]. RFA may be performed either intraoperatively or via a percutaneous approach, with a low morbidity rate in either case, although its role is still limited to selected patients [26].

Cytoreductive surgery limited to the primary tumor in patients with unresectable metastases is proposed in selected cases to alleviate mass-related symptoms by reducing tumor burden. Moreover, the analysis of retrospective series has demonstrated a measurable advantage in terms of survival after debulking [27] .

Liver transplantation is limited to 1% of patients. The main criteria for this approach include the presence of multiple metastases not amenable of other invasive procedures, the absence of extra-abdominal disease, a low Ki-67 value, and stable disease 1 year after diagnosis. Nevertheless, outcomes after transplantation for PanNEN liver metastases are heterogeneous and the efficacy of this strategy is still unclear [3].

10.2.5 Laparoscopic Approach for PanNENs

Both distal pancreatectomy and enucleation can be safely performed laparoscopically. The advantages of minimally invasive surgery are less postoperative pain, a better cosmetic result, a reduced length of hospital stay, and a faster postoperative recovery; the rate of pancreatic fistula formation is comparable to that observed after open surgery. It has been demonstrated that laparoscopic resections are safe and feasible in patients with presumed benign PanNENs whilst they are still a controversial procedure for those with malignancies. Whereas the laparoscopic approach is optimal for insulinomas and small non-functioning tumors, the role of laparoscopic surgery for gastrinomas is probably limited [28, 29].

10.3 PanNEN in Multiple Endocrine Neoplasia Type 1 (MEN1) Syndrome

Patients with MEN1 usually develop synchronous or metachronous PanNENs of various types: gastrinomas (54%), insulinomas (18%), and non-functional tumors (80–100%). The association of PanNENs with hereditary diseases such as MEN1 changes the surgical strategy due to the tendency towards disease multicentricity and the high rate of recurrence. To date, whereas surgery remains mandatory in case of tumor-related symptoms and a functioning tumor (e.g., insulinoma), the role of surgical treatment in small (< 2 cm) non-functioning PanNENs or gastrinomas is still unclear [30-32]. Small non-functioning PanNENs are commonly asymptomatic and their incidence is increasing due to better detection following the widespread use of modern cross-sectional imaging techniques. In MEN1 patients, only a few small tumors develop liver metastases or influence survival. Most recent studies suggests the active follow-up of small lesions and to operate only in the event of larger tumors (> 2 cm) and/or tumors growing or metastasizing during follow-up [32]. Similarly, since patients with small gastrinomas have excellent long-term survival also without surgical treatment and Zollinger–Ellison syndrome is easily controlled with medical treatment, surgery is commonly recommended only for lesion > 2 cm.

When surgery is indicated, the procedure ranges from enucleation to total pancreatectomy [6, 30]. The latter, although effective, is not generally recommended; instead, total pancreatectomy should be limited only to those patients in with multicentric lesions and a familial history of high mortality due to the disease. Enucleation is rarely the only needed procedure, mostly in small non-functioning PanNENs or benign functioning tumors such as insulinomas. Due to the high rate of multi-centric lesions, IOUS is always mandatory and it often leads to the decision to perform a subtotal distal pancreatectomy, with enucleation of those tumors located in the head of the pancreas or in the duodenal submucosa. When associated with an appropriate lymphadenectomy and duodenotomy for patients with suspected gastrinomas, the procedure is commonly called "Thompson's procedure." When a gastrinoma is associated, a pancreatico-duodenectomy generally results in a higher rate of cure (77–100%), although experience is poor since the procedure is rarely recommended [30, 33]. The associated high postoperative and long-term morbidity is commonly compared to the increasing evidence of good long-term survival (100% at 15 years) of patients with gastrinomas < 2 cm treated conservatively [31]. Pancreatico-duodenectomy may be advisable in patients with large tumors in the pancreatic head or duodenal tumor and in the presence of lymphadenopathy.

10.4　Conclusions

Despite recent advances in our understanding of neuroendocrine tumors, the appropriate surgical treatment of PanNENs remains challenging [34]. The optimal surgical strategy should be always tailored to the tumor's characteristics as well as the patient's symptoms, comorbidities, and life expectancy. Accordingly, these patients should be referred to highly experience centers in order to optimize the surgical indications and reduce operative morbidity. Moreover, proper communication with the patient and a multidisciplinary decision-making process are key elements in disease management, especially in advanced disease.

References

1. Rindi G, Kloppel G, Alhman H et al (2006) TNM staging of foregut (neuro)endocrine tumors: a consensus proposal including a grading system. Virchows Arch 449:395-401
2. Kulke MH, Anthony LB, Bushnell DL et al (2010) NANETS treatment guidelines: well-differentiated neuroendocrine tumors of the stomach and pancreas. Pancreas 39:735-752

10 Surgical Therapy

3. Falconi M, Bartsch DK, Eriksson B et al (2012) ENETS Consensus Guidelines for the Management of Patients with Digestive Neuroendocrine Neoplasms of the Digestive System: well-differentiated pancreatic non functioning tumors. Neuroendocrinology 95:120-134

4. Norton JA, Fraker DL, Alexander HR et al (1999) Surgery to cure the Zollinger-Ellison syndrome. N Engl J Med 341:635-644

5. Norton JA, Jensen RT (2004) Resolved and unresolved controversies in the surgical management of patients with Zollinger-Ellison syndrome. Ann Surg 240:757-773

6. Crippa S, Zerbi A, Boninsegna L et al (2012) Surgical management of insulinomas: short- and long-term outcomes after enucleations and pancreatic resections. Arch SurgMar 147:261-266

7. Norton JA (1994) Neuroendocrine tumors of the pancreas and duodenum. Curr Probl Surg 31:77-156

8. Falconi M, Plockinger U, Kwekkenboom DJ et al (2006) Well-differentiated pancreatic non-functioning tumors/carcinoma. Neuroendocrinology 84:196-211

9. Bettini R, Partelli S, Boninsegna L et al (Tumor size correlates with malignancy in nonfunctioning pancreatic endocrine tumor. Surgery 150:75-82

10. Falconi M, Zerbi A, Crippa S et al (2010) Parenchyma-preserving resections for small nonfunctioning pancreatic endocrine tumors. Ann Surg Oncol 17:1621-1627

11. Falconi M, Mantovani W, Crippa S et al (2008) Pancreatic insufficiency after different resections for benign tumors. Br J Surg 95:85-91

12. Aranha GV, Shoup M (2005) Nonstandard pancreatic resections for unusual lesions. Am J Surg 189:223-228

13. Boninsegna L, Panzuto F, Partelli S et al (2011) Malignant pancreatic neuroendocrine tumor: Lymph node ratio and Ki67 are predictors of recurrence after curative resections. Eur J Cancer [Epub ahead of print]

14. Akerstrom G, Hellman P (2007) Surgery on neuroendocrine tumors. Best Pract Res Clin Endocrinol Metab 21:87-109

15. Fendrich V, Langer P, Celik I et al (2006) An aggressive surgical approach leads to long-term survival in patients with pancreatic endocrine tumors. Ann Surg 244:845-851

16. Schurr PG, Strate T, Rese K et al (2007) Aggressive surgery improves long-term survival in neuroendocrine pancreatic tumors: an institutional experience. Ann Surg 245:273-281

17. Sutcliffe R, Maguire D, Ramage J et al (2004) Management of neuroendocrine liver metastases. Am J Surg 187:39-46

18. Chamberlain RS, Canes D, Brown KT et al (2000) Hepatic neuroendocrine metastases: does intervention alter outcomes? J Am Coll Surg 190:432-445

19. Chen H, Hardacre JM, Uzar A et al (1998) Isolated liver metastases from neuroendocrine tumors: does resection prolong survival? J Am Coll Surg 187:88-92

20. Sarmiento JM, Heywood G, Rubin J et al (2003) Surgical treatment of neuroendocrine metastases to the liver: a plea for resection to increase survival. J Am Coll Surg 197.29-37

21. Bettini R, Mantovani W, Boninsegna L et al (2009) Primary tumor resection in metastatic non-functioning pancreatic endocrine carcinomas. Dig Liver Dis 41:49-55

22. House MG, Cameron JL, Lillemoe KD et al (2006) Differences in survival for patients with resectable versus unresectable metastases from pancreatic islet cell cancer. J Gastrointest Surg 10:138-145

23. Touzios JG, Kiely JM, Pitt SC et al (2005) Neuroendocrine hepatic metastases: does aggressive management improve survival? Ann Surg 241:776-783

24. Yao KA, Talamonti MS, Nemcek A et al (2001) Indications and results of liver resection and hepatic chemoembolization for metastatic gastrointestinal neuroendocrine tumors. Surgery 130:677-682

25. Langergraber G, Gupta JK, Pressl A et al (2004) On-line monitoring for control of a pilot-scale sequencing batch reactor using a submersible UV/VIS spectrometer. Water Sci Technol 50:73-80

26. Mazzaglia PJ, Berber E, Milas M, Siperstein AE (2007) Laparoscopic radiofrequency ablation of neuroendocrine liver metastases: a 10-year experience evaluating predictors of survival. Surgery 142:10-19

27. Capurso G, Bettini R, Rinzivillo M et al (2011) Role of resection of the primary pancreatic neuroendocrine tumor only in patients with unresectable metastatic liver disease: a systematic review. Neuroendocrinology 93:223-229
28. Mabrut JY, Fernandez-Cruz L, Azagra JS et al (2005) Laparoscopic pancreatic resection: results of a multicenter European study of 127 patients. Surgery 137:597-605
29. Fernandez-Cruz L, Blanco L, Cosa R, Rendon H (2008) Is laparoscopic resection adequate in patients with neuroendocrine pancreatic tumors? World J Surg 32:904-917
30. Jensen RT, Berna MJ, Bingham DB, Norton JA (2008) Inherited pancreatic endocrine tumor syndromes: advances in molecular pathogenesis, diagnosis, management, and controversies. Cancer 113:1807-1843
31. Norton JA, Alexander HR, Fraker DL et al (2001) Comparison of surgical results in patients with advanced and limited disease with multiple endocrine neoplasia type 1 and Zollinger-Ellison syndrome. Ann Surg 234:495-505
32. Triponez F, Goudet P, Dosseh D et al (2006) Is surgery beneficial for MEN1 patients with small ≤ 2 cm), nonfunctioning pancreaticoduodenal endocrine tumor? An analysis of 65 patients from the GTE. World J Surg May 30:654-662
33. Lopez CL, Falconi M, Waldmann J et al (2012) Partial pancreaticoduodenectomy can provide cure for duodenal gastrinoma associated with multiple endocrine neoplasia type 1. Ann Surg [Epub ahead of print]
34. Rindi G, Falconi M, Klersy C et al (2012) TNM Staging of neoplasms of the endocrine pancreas: results from a large international cohort study. J Natl Cancer Inst 104:764-77

Functional Imaging and Peptide Receptor Radionuclide Therapy

11

Maria Chiara Ambrosetti, Duccio Volterrani, Federica Guidoccio, Lisa Bodei, Federica Orsini, Giuliano Mariani and Marco Ferdeghini

11.1 Introduction

Nuclear medicine imaging depicts the expression of certain target molecules and evaluates the functional aspects of lesions within tissues. The molecular information can be combined with the mainly anatomical information provided by other diagnostic modalities, e.g., conventional radiological imaging with ultrasonography (US), computed tomography (CT), magnetic resonance imaging (MRI), contrast-enhanced US (CEUS), endoscopic US (EUS), intraoperative US (IOUS), and selective angiography with hormonal sampling. Thus, nuclear medicine imaging can identify specific molecular changes linked to the target expression of macroscopic lesions within tissues.

Neuroendocrine neoplasms (NENs) are characterized by the presence of receptors for somatostatin (SSTR) and/or for other hormone-like peptides on the cell membrane, and/or by the presence of neuroamine uptake mechanisms. Six subtypes of SSTR have been identified by molecular analysis ($sstr_1$, $sstr_{2a}$, $sstr_{2b}$, $sstr_3$, $sstr_4$, and $sstr_5$). Each receptor exerts its action by inhibiting adenylyl cyclase activity. SSTR density is markedly elevated in malignant neuroendocrine cells (from 80 to 2000 fmol/mg protein), while SSTR expression is relatively low within normal neuroendocrine tissues [1]. NENs can also have the property of taking up amino acids and transforming them into biogenic amines by means of decarboxylation; for instance, they can convert the amino acid tyrosine into L-DOPA, which is subsequently decarboxylated to dopamine, oxidated to norepinephrine, and methylated to yield epinephrine, which is accumulated in pre-synaptic vesicles. The expression of membrane

---

M. Federghini (✉)
Department of Pathology and Diagnostics, Radiology Unit, "G.B. Rossi" University Hospital, Verona, Italy
e-mail: marco.federghini@univr.it

P. Pederzoli and C. Bassi (eds.), *Uncommon Pancreatic Neoplasms*,
Updates in Surgery
DOI: 10.1007/978-88-470-2673-5_11, © Springer-Verlag Italia 2013

transporters, enzymes, and the neurosecretory vesicles for catecholamines constitute the pathophysiologic background for radionuclide imaging of transformation.

Finally, since the high glucose metabolism of tumors is directly related to cell proliferation (depending on the genetic expression of glucose transporters, GLUT), the capability of NEN cells to accumulate the radiopharmaceutical [^{18}F]FDG typically is related to cell dedifferentiation and high biological aggressiveness, as typically observed in the most malignant forms of NENs.

11.2 Radiopharmaceuticals

Over the last 20 years the use of radiolabeled somatostatin analogues as high-affinity tracers for specific binding to SSTRs has allowed successful gamma-camera functional imaging of NENs, initially with single-photon-emitting radiopharmaceuticals (using conventional gamma cameras), then also with positron-emitting radiopharmaceuticals (using positron emission tomography, PET). In this regard, whole-body somatostatin receptor scintigraphy (SRS) has revolutionized the diagnostic and therapeutic approach to patients with NENs.

All radiopharmaceuticals currently in use for imaging SSTR-positive neoplasms are based on octreotide, a long-acting 8-amino acid analog of the native 14- or 28-amino acid human peptide hormone somatostatin (Fig. 11.1);

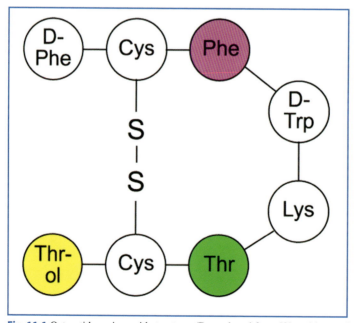

Fig. 11.1 Octreotide amino acid structure. (Reproduced from [2], with permission)

in fact, native somatostatin has an extremely short plasma half-life, which limits the ability to detect its specific tissue accumulation following systemic administration. Octreotide binds to sstr$_2$ with high affinity (K_d 0.1–1 nM), whereas it exhibits a moderate affinity (within the 10–100 nM range) for sstr$_3$ and sstr$_5$, and a very low affinity for sstr$_1$ and sstr$_4$.

The presence of octreotide-binding SSTRs on NENs allows the in vivo functional visualization of these tumors with the use of radiolabeled somatostatin analogues. ^{123}I-[Tyr^3]-octreotide was the first radiotracer developed for this purpose. However, its clinical application was limited by the relatively high background radioactivity in the abdomen and by its relatively short half-life, both in physical terms (13 h for ^{123}I) and in biological terms (fast dehalogenation in vivo). ^{111}In-[DTPA D-Phe]-octreotide, or ^{111}In-pentetreotide, has instead been widely used and is still employed for the clinical assessment of NENs, because of its better in-vivo stability and the fact that the longer physical half-life of ^{111}In allows scintigraphic imaging also at relatively delayed times after administration (up to at least 24 h post-injection). It is a registered trademark of Mallinckrodt Inc., under the name of Octreoscan.

A number of ^{99m}Tc-labeled somatostatin analogues have more recently been developed (e.g., ^{99m}Tc-depreotide, ^{99m}Tc-vapreotide, ^{99m}Tc-P829), considering that, for gamma-camera imaging, the photon emission of ^{99m}Tc is more suitable than that of ^{111}In. Particularly promising is ^{99m}Tc-EDDA-HYNIC-TOC in the imaging of sst$_{2/5}$-positive tumors, as it is superior to ^{111}In-pentetreotide [3, 4]. Nevertheless, the development of PET tracers has prompted a totally new era in receptor imaging of NENs, further modifying the diagnostic work-up for the assessment of these tumors.

Single-photon imaging with radio-iodinated meta-iodobenzylguanidine ([^{123}I]MIBG) and PET imaging with [^{18}F]-DOPA or [^{18}F]-dopamine are highly sensitive in the detection of tumors arising from the adrenal medulla; these compounds are also taken up by non-adrenomedullary pancreatic NENs (PanNENs), which sometimes express transporters and neurosecretory vesicles for catecholamines (Fig. 11.2).

More recently, the use of ^{68}Ga-labeled somatostatin analogues has further expanded the nuclear medicine armamentarium, such that advanced PET/CT imaging of NENs allows their molecular/functional characterization. ^{68}Ga-labeled somatostatin analogues consist of a somatostatin-like peptidic structure that actively binds SSTRs, together with a chelant (DOTA) and the positron-emitting radionuclide (^{68}Ga). Most clinical experience so far accumulated has been obtained with three radiolabeled peptides: ^{68}Ga-DOTA-TOC (1,4,7,10-tetraazacyclododecane,1,4,7,10-tetraacetic acid Tyr^3 octreotide), ^{68}Ga-DOTA-NOC (1,4,7,10-tetraazacyclododecane,1,4,7,10-tetraacetic acid 1-Nal^3 octreotide), resulting from an amino acid exchange at position 3 of octreotide, and ^{68}Ga-DOTA-TATE (1,4,7,10-tetraazacyclododecane,1,4,7,10-tetraacetic acid Thr^8 octreotide). In ^{68}Ga-DOTA-NOC there is a simple amino acid substitution in position 3 of octreotide, while in ^{68}Ga-DOTA-TATE a carboxylic acid group replaces the alcohol group at the C-terminus of the peptide,

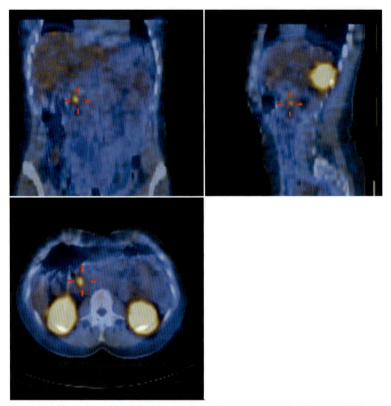

Fig. 11.2 ^{123}I-MIBG SPECT/CT in a patient with a pancreatic insulinoma. While prior scintigraphy with Octreoscan was negative, the ^{123}I-MIBG scan clearly visualized the tumor, located in the head of the pancreas. (Reproduced from [2], with permission)

resulting in the formation of DOTA-D-Phe^1-Tyr^3-Thr^8-octreotide. All three bind with high affinity to sstr$_2$ and sstr$_5$, while DOTA-NOC has good affinity also for sstr$_3$ [5, 6]. The binding affinity of ^{68}Ga-DOTA-TATE for sstr$_2$ is considerably higher than that of ^{111}In-DTPA-octreotide, while its binding affinity for sstr$_5$ is lower; for sstr$_3$, it has negligible affinity and for sstr$_1$ and sst4$_4$ little or none [7, 8].

The labeling procedure of ^{68}Ga-DOTA-peptides is easily and quickly carried out at an on-site radiochemical laboratory, with relatively low overall costs. In fact, ^{68}Ga can be eluted from commercially available ^{68}Ge/^{68}Ga generators, which can be used for approximately 9–12 months because of the long physical half-life (270.8 days) of the mother radionuclide ^{68}Ge. ^{68}Ga (with a physical half-life of 68 min) has an 89% positron emission and a 3.2% gamma emission (1077 keV). The ^{68}Ga eluate is first concentrated and purified using a micro-chromatography method [9], with peptide labeling subsequently achieved within 15 min, with a > 95% yield.

11.3 Nuclear Medicine Imaging of PanNENs

Soon after its introduction into clinical practice, Octreoscan imaging was reported to be very useful for patients with NENs as it explores the whole body and provides important clinical indications, allowing the accurate detection and localization of the primary tumor based on its expression of SSTRs. Moreover, this imaging technique provides valuable information for staging disease extent, for identifying metastases to soft tissue or bone, and for restaging NEN patients during follow-up. In this regard, it should be emphasized that SRS (with either single-photon or positron emitting radiopharmaceuticals) cannot be considered as a true "diagnostic" procedure, i.e., for differentiating NENs from other tumors; in fact, several other types of tumors can also express SSTRs with high density, besides the possibility of SSTR expression also in benign lesions (e.g., chronic granulomatous diseases). The diagnosis of NENs is mostly based on clinical/biochemical findings, while imaging plays an important role for localizing the disease site(s), which is not an easy task even with high-resolution imaging techniques such as CT and/or MRI for tumors that can be very small and distributed virtually throughout the entire body. Thus, the main role of SRS in the initial approach to patients with a newly diagnosed NEN is its ability to localize the exact site(s) of the tumor(s), also as a possible guide for surgical resection.

Nuclear medicine imaging of NENs is crucial for planning therapy also in patients with non-resectable lesions; in fact, the tumor expression and density of SSTRs can guide therapeutic decision-making in NEN patients, by identifying those who will benefit from therapy with "cold" vs. radiolabeled somatostatin analogues as well as those who are candidates for chemo-radiotherapy.

SRS with Octreoscan is highly sensitive for the detection and staging of PanNENs. In general, gastrinomas abundantly express SSTRs; in particular, about 50% of gastrinomas express $sstr_2$ and $sstr_5$, 33% express $sstr_1$, 17% express $sstr_3$, and 83% express $sstr_4$ [10]. Whole-body SRS has a pivotal role in these NENs [11, 12], identifying with 60–90% sensitivity both the primary lesion and metastases [13, 14]. However, few studies have been published supporting the usefulness of SRS in patients with somatostatinomas. Although some authors [15] reported that these tumors can be SSTR-negative in binding assays and in receptor autoradiography experiments (mainly because the high levels of circulating somatostatin induce receptor down-regulation), in vivo visualization of somatostatinomas with SRS has been reported to be effective both within the pancreas and at distant metastatic sites [16].

Among the SSTRr receptors, $sstr_2$ is expressed in 100% of the patients with glucagonomas, while $sstr_1$, $sstr_3$, $sstr_4$, and $sstr_5$ are expressed in approximately two-thirds [10]. In these patients, SRS has a sensitivity of approximately 70% for primary tumor detection and distant staging. Since most pancreatic VIPomas express all five SSTR subtypes [10], SRS in these patients (who usually present with a large tumor in the tail of the pancreas) is useful for lesion localization and characterization, and for the detection of distant metastases.

The overall sensitivity of SRS is about 86%, being much lower, as expected, for lesions < 1 cm in size [17].

Insulinomas often present as a small lesion characterized by low $sstr_2$ expression [18]. About 50% of these tumors express $sstr_1$, while 15–20% express $sstr_3$ and $sstr_4$ [19]. Therefore the sensitivity of SRS for insulinomas can be as low as 50–60% [13, 20]. Although non-malignant insulinomas rarely express SSTRs, in malignant insulinomas functional evaluation with SRS is highly recommended for tumor detection and staging as well as for determining the indications for therapy based on somatostatin analogs [21]. Secondary insulinomas often have higher $sstr_2$ expression than the primary tumor [13, 22, 23].

In the initial approach to patients with newly diagnosed PanNENs, the integration of SRS data with those provided by anatomic imaging is crucial. Due to the recent introduction into clinical routine of SPECT/CT hybrid equipment, radionuclide imaging can now provide the surgeon with detailed functional and topographic information for tissue sampling and resectability; in addition, it can exclude false-positive findings due to accessory spleen, recent surgical scars, and any other cause of granulomatous-lymphoid infiltrate that may mimic a tumor. Moreover, correlative imaging can aid the nuclear physician in correctly identifying small lesions that might have reduced SSTR expression because of recent treatments, as well as de-differentiated disease, both of which may lead to false-negative results at SRS (Fig. 11.3).

The diagnostic impact of SRS is mainly during initial staging, as the technique has been shown to modify the therapeutic strategy in up to 53% of patients with NENs. In fact, because of its high sensitivity in detecting distant metastases (61–96%), SRS may prevent surgery with curative intent in those patients whose tumors have already metastasized [24, 25]. Moreover, SRS is the most accurate imaging modality for the "one-shot" detection of liver and extrahepatic metastases in patients with pancreatic NENs (Fig. 11.4), although sensitivity can be adversely affected by the small size typical of metastatic lesions.

SRS also may be useful in the follow-up of patients, in particular to monitor the efficacy of treatment. In this regard, changes in functional volume have been reported to be more reliable than RECIST (Response Evaluation Criteria in Solid Tumors) and correlate well with the long-term clinical response [26]. Moreover, SRS can aid in the identification of potentially responsive patients for treatment with unlabeled somatostatin analogues (such as octreotide acetate), or with tumor-targeted somatostatin analogues radiolabeled with either ^{90}Y or ^{177}Lu. In the former approach, it is still debated whether the sensitivity of SRS is reduced in patients concurrently receiving therapeutic doses of octreotide acetate; thus, consideration should be given to temporarily suspending therapy before administering the radiopharmaceutical.

As alluded to above, the introduction of receptor PET radiopharmaceuticals has prompted a new era in receptor imaging for NENs. Based on its unique pharmacokinetics, ^{68}Ga-DOTA-TOC achieves high tumor/non-tumor ratios

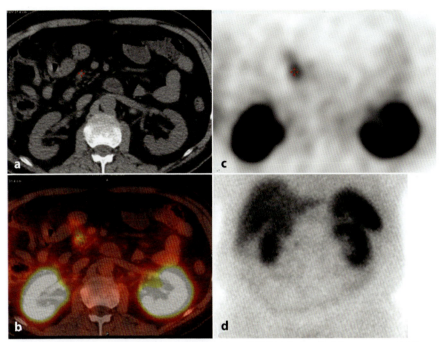

Fig. 11.3 Octreoscan examination in a patient with an NEN in the head of the pancreas. (**a**) Low-dose CT image, (**b**) trans-axial SPECT image, (**c**) fused hybrid Octreoscan SPECT/CT CT imaging. While planar imaging revealed only faint uptake (**d**), SPECT/CT imaging clearly improved visualization of the tumor

within a short period after its administration and is even better than DOTA-TOC containing other metal ions. In particular, 80% of the activity is accumulated in the tumors within 30 min, renal clearance is fast, and the radioactivity concentration in tissues not expressing SSTRs is very low. The combination of high contrast and fast imaging, as well as the better spatial resolution of PET compared with single-photon imaging allows the detection of smaller lesions not identified at SRS; this feature becomes of paramount importance in tailoring the clinical management of NENs on a patient-to-patient basis [27]. Moreover, the ability of PET to accurately quantify uptake in each lesion (in terms of SUV) allows the use of such data for monitoring the response to therapy. Finally, PET imaging with ^{68}Ga-DOTA-somatostatin analogues involves less radiation exposure for the patient than is the case for imaging with ^{111}In-pentetreotide.

Current data show that, despite some differences in receptor binding affinity among the three different ^{68}Ga-DOTA-somatostatin analogues (-TOC, -NOC, -TATE), there is no direct clinical correlate regarding advantages in the clinical accuracy of one radiopharmaceutical over the others. All of them have in fact been reported to provide clinically accurate and valuable information

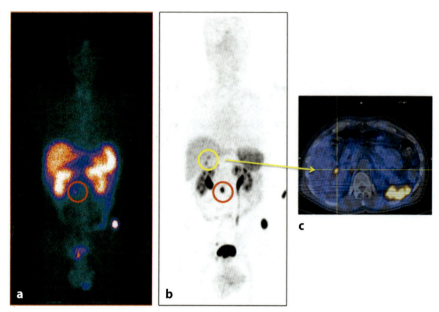

Fig. 11.4 Comparison between Octreoscan (**a** whole-body planar image) and ^{68}Ga-DOTA-TOC PET/CT (**b** MIP and **c** trans-axial fused PET/CT images). Liver metastases were detected only by ^{68}Ga- DOTA-TOC PET/CT. (Image courtesy of Prof. Stefano Fanti, Nuclear Medicine Service, "S. Orsola" University Hospital, Bologna, Italy)

for NEN imaging, as consistently demonstrated by high tumor/non-tumor ratios, and definitely higher sensitivity than SRS [28]. Moreover, ^{68}Ga-DOTA-TOC and ^{68}Ga-DOTA-TATE can mimic as closely as possible the in vivo pharmacokinetic patterns of their ^{90}Y- or ^{177}Lu-labeled counterparts used for peptide receptor radionuclide therapy (PRRT) [29].

^{68}Ga-DOTA-peptide PET performs better than CT and/or single-photon SRS for locating well-differentiated NEN lesions, accurately detecting even small-sized tumors, in particular metastatic sites in lymph nodes or bone [30] or tumors with unusual anatomical locations [31]. However, it should be underlined that the detection of a greater number of lesions does not always impact disease stage or the therapeutic approach.

In 84 patients with NEN, ^{68}Ga-DOTA-TOC PET/CT was reported to have 97% sensitivity for the detection of SSTR-positive lesions, superior to both CT (61%) and single-photon SRS (52%) [32]. In another series of 51 patients with well-differentiated NEN, ^{68}Ga-DOTA-TOC showed 97% sensitivity and 92% specificity in the early detection of bone metastases, much higher than CT and SRS [33].

Staging, clinical management, and the therapeutic approach can be changed when unsuspected metastatic disease or local relapse is identified, or SSTR expression on NEN cells by ^{68}Ga-DOTA-peptides is confirmed/excluded, unlike conventional imaging. In 50 out of 90 NEN patients, ^{68}Ga-DOTA-NOC PET/CT was reported to impact the therapeutic approach with PRRT or with unlabeled somatostatin analogue treatment in 36 patients, surgical treatment in six patients; surgical treatment was excluded in another six patients, radiotherapy in one patient, liver transplantation in one patient, and further diagnostic assessment in one patient [34]. In 51 patients with NENs, 35 with negative and 16 with equivocal ^{111}In-DTPA-octreotide uptake on SRS, ^{68}Ga-DOTA-TATE PET detected significantly more lesions than SRS and modified management in 70.6% of the patients, subsequently considered candidates for PRRT [35].

Non-invasive quantification of the receptor expression pattern is especially useful for selecting those patients eligible for targeted therapy with either radiolabeled or cold somatostatin analogs as the most appropriate therapeutic approach. High uptake of ^{68}Ga-DOTA-peptides reflects a high SSTR expression on well-differentiated NENs, associated with slower growth rate and a higher likelihood of response to targeted therapy with either hot or cold somatostatin analogs. The SUV_{max} derived from ^{68}Ga-DOTA-NOC PET/CT has recently been reported to be a helpful prognostic factor of outcome in this regard. Out of 44 patients with NENs, the SUV_{max} was significantly higher in those with stable disease/partial response and provided valuable information to distinguish those patients showing progressive disease at follow-up. In particular, an $SUV_{max} > 19.3$ allowed the selection of patients with slower disease progression [35]. Although there is no agreement on the use of ^{68}Ga-DOTA-peptides for assessing response to PRRT [31], they are widely employed to quantify the presence of SSTRs, radiopharmaceutical biodistribution prior to treatment [36], and to predict and assess the response to peptide receptor therapies in NENs.

Compared with MIBG scintigraphy, radiolabeled somatostatin analogues have been shown to be more accurate for detecting gastro-entero-pancreatic NENs and their metastases. Similar results have been observed with [^{18}F]DOPA PET. In patients with well-differentiated NEN, ^{68}Ga-DOTA-TATE showed marginally higher sensitivity than ^{18}F-DOPA (96% vs. 56%) [37].

Preoperative localization of the lesions in patients with congenital hyperinsulinism is currently the only application of [^{18}F]DOPA PET in pancreatic malignancy. Hyperfunctioning pancreatic lesions have greater L-DOPA uptake and conversion to dopamine than normally functioning pancreatic tissue, which expresses only low levels of aromatic amino acid decarboxylase. The high sensitivity of this imaging approach could allow mini-invasive laparoscopic surgery with limited resections, reducing therefore the risk of long-term diabetes [38]. On the other hand, euglycemic and hyperinsulinemic adult patients show [^{18}F]DOPA uptake in the whole pancreas, the main limitation for identifying insulinomas or β-cell hyperplasia.

Several papers have demonstrated that NENs with a positive [^{18}F]FDG PET have increased aggressiveness, irrespective of either grading or the Ki67 proliferation index [39]. In fact, high glucose metabolism of tumors depending on

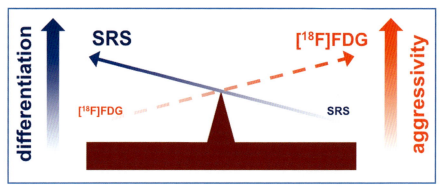

Fig. 11.5 "Flip-flop" pattern of neuroendocrine tumors. Higher ^{18}[F]FDG uptake combined with lower Octreoscan uptake correlates with higher disease aggressiveness (and vice versa)

increased GLUT expression is directly related to cell proliferation and failed differentiation [40]. The dedifferentiation of neoplastic NEN cells typically tends to increase their uptake of [^{18}F]FDG. Thus, a high glucose metabolic state can provide crucial prognostic information (Fig. 11.5).

^{68}Ga-DOTA-TOC has been reported to detect a higher number of tumors in well-differentiated NENs than is the case with [^{18}F]FDG [41]. Compared with [^{18}F]FDG PET/CT, ^{68}Ga-DOTA-TATE PET/CT has higher uptake by well-differentiated, low-grade NENs. [^{18}F]FDG does not provide valuable information in the assessment of well-differentiated, relatively slow growing NENs, characterized by a low metabolic rate and therefore low glucose consumption. Instead, it has an important role in higher grade, poorly differentiated NENs, which have a high fraction of proliferating cells (positive Ki-67 staining in > 5% of cells); furthermore, for lesions with low SSTR expression [^{18}F]FDG PET better demonstrates progression on morphological imaging over a period of < 6 months [42] than either CT or MRI.

Therefore, the use of radiopharmaceuticals with different mechanism(s) of uptake, i.e., an SSTR tracer (^{68}Ga-DOTA-peptides) and a metabolic tracer ([^{18}F]FDG), may provide more accurate information on tumor biology, and thus more accurate patient management. Detecting the presence of undifferentiated areas/lesions with high glucose metabolism has a relevant impact in the selection of standard chemotherapy over PRRT.

11.4 Peptide Receptor Radionuclide Therapy

PRRT is a new modality that uses radiolabeled peptides for treating unresectable or metastasized NENs. The rationale for such therapy is to convey radioactivity inside the tumor cells, where sensitive targets, such as DNA, can be hit as a result of internalization of the somatostatin receptor and radiolabeled analogue complex.

Several peptides labeled with therapeutic radiometals, such as ^{90}Y or ^{177}Lu, have been explored for therapeutic purposes. Among these, ^{90}Y-DOTA-TOC and ^{177}Lu-DOTA-TATE are the most widely employed radiopeptides. The choice of these two particular molecules derives from pharmacokinetic considerations. The pharmacokinetic profiles of DOTA-TOC and DOTA-TATE are particularly favorable, with a rapid plasma clearance after administration and a relevant renal excretion (about 70% of the injected dose in urine after 24 h) [43, 44]. ^{90}Y has a higher β-particle emission than ^{177}Lu. Based on an analysis of the residence times for DOTA-TATE and DOTA-TOC, ^{177}Lu has greater advantages when labeling DOTA-TATE, while in view of the higher renal dose from ^{177}Lu-DOTA-TATE, ^{90}Y is better in the labeling of DOTA-TOC.

Tumor candidates for PRRT with radiolabeled somatostatin analogs are basically sstr$_2$-expressing NENs, and SRS is currently the most accurate and validated method to assess the presence of SSTR overexpression. The absorbed dose depends on the activity residing in the tumor and on its mass. With equal amounts of radioactivity accumulation, smaller masses have higher chances of volume reduction, due to a higher absorbed dose. This is confirmed by clinical data evaluating the response to therapy in relatively large groups of patients: those with a limited volume of liver metastases responded to PRRT, while those with a high tumor load did not [45].

PRRT with either ^{90}Y-DOTA-TOC or ^{177}Lu-DOTA-TATE is generally well tolerated, without serious acute side effects. Due to their radiosensitivity at the cumulative activities normally reached, the kidneys are the critical organs in PRRT, particularly after ^{90}Y-DOTA-TOC administration. The administration of L-lysine and/or L-arginine in order to competitively inhibit proximal tubular re-absorption of the radiopeptide can reduce the renal dose by 9–53% [46-48]. A median 7.3% decline in creatinine clearance per year was reported after ^{90}Y-DOTA-TOC therapy, compared to 3.8% per year after ^{177}Lu-DOTA-TATE. Cumulative and per-cycle renal absorbed dose, patient age, the presence of hypertension, and diabetes are factors contributing to the decline of renal function after PRRT [49]. Kidney radiation toxicity is typically evident several months after irradiation, due to the slow repair properties of renal cells.

Fertility can be temporarily impaired in men undergoing PRRT, due to radiation damage to Sertoli cells. Finally, it must be considered that treating functioning NENs with PRRT may result in acute cell rupture and hence the exacerbation of clinical syndromes (such as hypoglycemia, carcinoid, or Zollinger-Ellison syndromes), sometimes severely to the extent that further hospitalization and adequate care are required [50, 51].

Dosimetry estimates for normal organs and malignant lesions are a fundamental aid in planning PRRT, in order to deliver the maximum dose to the tumor while remaining within the therapeutic window with respect to the dose delivered to the normal organs, particularly the kidney (the dose limiting organ) and the bone marrow. Individual pre-therapeutic dosimetry is necessary for patient selection and therapy planning, because there are enormous differences amongst patients regarding radiopeptide uptake in normal organs and in tumor tissues.

The radiopeptide that has been most extensively studied for PRRT is ^{90}Y-DOTA-TOC. Despite differences in clinical phase I–II protocols from various centers, complete and partial remissions have been recorded in 10–30% of patients. In a first report, 29 patients were treated with a dose-escalating scheme consisting of four or more cycles of ^{90}Y-DOTA-TOC with cumulative activities of 6.12 ± 1.35 GBq/m^2. Twenty of these patients showed disease stabilization, two had partial remission, four minor remission, and three had disease progression [52]. Although patients with pancreatic NENs had an objective response rate of 38%, a significant reduction of clinical symptoms was observed in the majority of the patients treated [53]. Toxicity was generally mild and involved the kidney and bone marrow.

Genuine phase II studies with ^{90}Y-DOTA-TOC are still lacking, but experiences in selected series of patients, mostly retrospective, have been reported in the literature. A tentative categorization of the objective response according to tumor type was attempted in a meta-analysis of results in GEP tumors. PanNENs were the tumors that better responded to PRRT [54]. According to this review, the results obtained with [^{90}Y-DOTA^0,Tyr^3]octreotide and [^{177}Lu-DOTA^0,Tyr^3]octreotate are very encouraging. There are several reasons that might explain a certain variability in the rate of tumor responses observed after PRRT with [^{90}Y-DOTA^0,Tyr^3]octreotide: (a) the administered activities vary both in terms of total administered dose and schedule of treatment (single cycle vs. multiple cycles, dose-escalating protocols vs. fixed activities, etc.); (b) differences between patients as well as tumor characteristics; (c) degree of uptake on Octreoscan imaging; (c) estimated total tumor burden; (d) extent of liver involvement.

Therefore, differences in patient selection play an important role in determining treatment outcome; however, a direct, randomized comparison of the various treatments is still lacking (Table 11.1). Figure 11.6 provides an example of an objective response to ^{90}Y-DOTA-TOC therapy in a patient with gross liver metastases from a pancreatic insulinoma treated with 23 GBq administered in seven sequential cycles.

11 Functional Imaging and Peptide Receptor Radionuclide Therapy

Table 11.1 Tumor responses to PRRT in patients with gastro-entero-pancreatic (GEP) NENs treated with different radiolabeled somatostatin analogues

Reference Group	Ligand	No. of patients	Tumor response					
			CR[a]	PR[a]	MR[a]	SD[a]	PD[a]	CR + PR[b]
Rotterdam	[^{111}In-DTPA^0]octreotide	26	0	0	5 (19)	11 (42)	10 (38)	0
New Orleans	[^{111}In-DTPA^0]octreotide	26	0	2 (8)	NA	21 (81)	3 (12)	8
Milan	[^{90}Y-DOTA^0, Tyr^3]octreotide	21	0	6 (29)	NA	11 (52)	4 (19)	29
Basel	[^{90}Y-DOTA^0, Tyr^3]octreotide	74	3 (4)	15 (20)	NA	48 (65)	8 (11)	24
Basel	[^{90}Y-DOTA^0, Tyr^3]octreotide	33	2 (6)	9 (27)	NA	19 (57)	3 (9)	33
Rotterdam	[^{90}Y-DOTA^0, Tyr^3]octreotide	54	0	4 (7)	7 (13)	33 (61)	10 (19)	7
Rotterdam	[^{177}Lu-DOTA^0, Tyr^3]octreotate	76	1 (1)	22 (29)	9 (12)	30 (39)	14 (18)	30

CR, complete response; *PR*, partial response; *MR*, minor response; *SD*, stable disease; *PD*, progressive disease; *NA*, not available.
[a]Reported as number (percentage) of patients.
[b]Reported as percentage of patients.

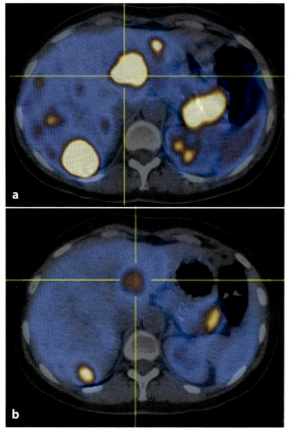

Fig. 11.6 ^{68}Ga-DOTA-TOC trans-axial PET/CT images obtained before (**a**) and after (**b**) PRRT with ^{90}Y-DOTA-TOC for treatment of liver metastatic involvement in a patient with pancreatic insulinoma

References

1. Wong F, Kim E (2001) Peptide receptor imaging, In Kim E, Yang D (eds) Targeted molecular imaging in oncology, Springer Verlag, New York, Berlin, Heidelberg, pp. 102-110
2. Guidoccio F, Borsò E, Volterrani D (2010) Tecniche diagnostiche per lo studio dei tumori neuroendocrini. In: Volterrani D, Erba PA, Mariani G (eds.) Fondamenti di Medicina Nucleare - Tecniche e Applicazioni. Springer, Milan, pp. 681-692
3. Virgolini I (2000) Peptide imaging. Springer, Berlin, Heidelberg, New York
4. Lebtahi R, Le Cloirec J, Houzard C et al (2002) Detection of neuroendocrine tumors: ^{99m}Tc-P829 scintigraphy compared with ^{111}In-pentetreotide scintigraphy. J Nucl Med 43:889-895
5. Wild D, Schmitt JS, Ginj M et al (2003) DOTANOC, a high-affinity ligand of somatostatin receptor subtypes 2, 3 and 5 for labelling with various radiometals. Eur J Nucl Med Mol Imaging 30:1338-1347
6. Antunes P, Ginj M, Zhang H et al (2007) Are radiogallium-labelled DOTA-conjugated somatostatin analogues superior to those labelled with other radiometals? Eur J Nucl Med Mol Imaging 34:982-993
7. Kwekkeboom D, Bakker WH, Kooij PP et al (2001) ^{177}Lu-DOTA^{0}Tyr^3-octreotate: comparison with ^{111}In-DTPA^0-octreotide in patients. Eur J Nucl Med 28:1319-1325

8. Reubi JC, Schar JC, Waser B et al (2000) Affinity profiles for human somatostatin receptor subtypes SST_1-SST_5 of somatostatin radiotracers selected for scintigraphic and radiotherapeutic use. Eur J Nucl Med 27:273–282

9. Zhernosekov KP, Filosofov DV, Baum RP et al (2007) Processing of generator-produced ^{68}Ga for medical application. J Nucl Med 48:1741-1748

10. Oberg K (2004) Future aspects of somatostatin-receptor-mediated therapy. Neuroendocrinology 80:57–61

11. Plockinger U, Rindi G, Arnold R et al (2004) Guidelines for the diagnosis and treatment of neuroendocrine gastrointestinal tumours. A consensus statement on behalf of the European Neuroendocrine Tumour Society (ENETS). Neuroendocrinology 80:394-424

12. Modlin IM, Oberg K, Chung DC et al (2008) Gastroenteropancreatic neuroendocrine tumours. Lancet Oncology 9:61-72

13. Krenning EP, Kwekkeboom DJ, Bakker WH et al (1993) Somatostatin receptor scintigraphy with ^{111}In-DTPA-D-Phe[1]- and ^{123}I-Tyr[3].-octreotide: the Rotterdam experience with more than 1000 patients. Eur J Nucl Med 20:716-731

14. Gibril F, Doppman JL, Reynolds JC et al (1998) Bone metastases in patients with gastrinomas: a prospective study of bone scanning, somatostatin receptor scanning, and magnetic resonance image in their detection, frequency, location, and effect of their detection on management. J Clin Oncol 16:1040-1053

15. Reubi JC, Waser B, Lamberts SW, Mengod G (1993) Somatostatin (SRIH) messenger ribonucleic acid expression in human neuroendocrine and brain tumors using in situ hybridization histochemistry: comparison with SRIH receptor content. J Clin Endocrinol Metab 76:642-647

16. Schillaci O, Annibale B, Scopinaro F et al (2000) Somatostatin receptor scintigraphy of malignant somatostatinoma with indium-111-pentetreotide. J Nucl Med 38:886-887

17. Thomason JW, Martin RS, Fincher ME (2000) Somatostatin receptor scintigraphy: the definitive technique for characterizing vasoactive intestinal peptide-secreting tumors. Clin Nucl Med 25:661-664

18. Kwekkeboom DJ, Krenning EP, Scheidhauer K et al (2009) ENETS Consensus Guidelines for the Standards of Care in Neuroendocrine Tumors: somatostatin receptor imaging with ^{111}In-pentetreotide. Neuroendocrinology 90:184-189

19. Bertherat J, Tenenbaum F, Perlemoine K et al (2003) Somatostatin receptors 2 and 5 are the major somatostatin receptors in insulinomas: an in vivo and in vitro study. J Clin Endocrinol Metab 88:5353-5360

20. Virgolini I, Traub-Weidinger T, Decristoforo C (2005) Nuclear medicine in the detection and management of pancreatic islet cell tumours. Best Pract Res Clin Endocrinol Metab 19:213-227

21. Proye C, Malvaux P, Pattou F (1998) Non-invasive imaging of insulinomas and gastrinomas with endoscopic ultrasonography and somatostatin receptor scintigraphy. Surgery 124:1134-1144

22. Jamar F, Fiasse R, Leners N et al (1995) Somatostatin receptor imaging with indium-111-pentetreotide in gastro-enteropancreatic neuroendocrine tumors: safety, efficacy and impact on patient management. J Nucl Med 36:542-549

23. Gibril F, Jensen RT (2004) Diagnostic uses of radiolabelled somatostatin receptor analogues in gastroentero-pancreatic endocrine tumours. Dig Liver Dis 36:S106-120

24. Schillaci O, Spanu A, Scopinaro F et al (2003) Somatostatin receptor scintigraphy in liver metastasis detection from gastroenteropancreatic neuroendocrine tumors. J Nucl Med 44:359-368

25. Perri M, Erba P, Volterrani D et al (2008) Octreo-SPECT/CT imaging for accurate detection and localization of suspected neuroendocrine tumors. Q J Nucl Med Mol Imaging 52:323-333

26. Gopinath G, Ahmed A, Buscombe JR et al (2004) Prediction of clinical outcome in treated neuroendocrine tumours of carcinoid type using functional volumes on ^{111}In-pentetreotide SPECT imaging. Nucle Med Commun 25:253-257

27. Hofmann M, Maecke H, Borner R et al (2001) Biokinetics and imaging with the somatostatin receptor PET radioligand ^{68}Ga-DOTATOC: preliminary data. Eur J Nucl Med 28:1751-1777
28. Kowalski J, Henze M, Schuhmacher J et al (2003) Evaluation of positron emission tomography imaging using ^{68}Ga-DOTAD Phe^1-Tyr^3-Octreotide in comparison to ^{111}In-DTPAOC SPECT - First results in patients with neuro-endocrine tumors. Mol Imaging Biol 5:42-48
29. Kwekkeboom DJ, Kam BL, van Essen M et al (2010) Somatostatin receptor-based imaging and therapy of gastroenteropancreatic neuroendocrine tumors. Endocrine-Related Cancer 17:R53-73
30. Ambrosini V, Tomassetti P, Castellucci P et al (2008) Comparison between ^{68}Ga-DOTA-NOC and ^{18}F-DOPA PET for the detection of gastro-enteropancreatic and lung neuroendocrine tumours. Eur J Nucl Med Mol Imaging 35:1431-1438
31. Fanti S, Ambrosini V, Tomassetti P et al (2008) Evaluation of unusual neuroendocrine tumours by means of ^{68}Ga-DOTA-NOC PET. Biomed Pharmacother 62:667-771
32. Gabriel M, Decristoforo C, Kendler D et al (2007) ^{68}Ga-DOTA-Tyr^3-octreotide PET in neuroendocrine tumors: comparison with somatostatin receptor scintigraphy and CT. J Nucl Med 48:508-518
33. Putzer D, Gabriel M, Henninger B et al (2009) Bone metastases in patients with neuroendocrine tumor: ^{68}Ga-DOTA-Tyr^3-octreotide PET in comparison to CT and bone scintigraphy. J Nucl Med 50:1214-1221
34. Ambrosini V, Campana D, Bodei L et al (2010) ^{68}Ga-DOTANOC PET/CT clinical impact in patients with neuroendocrine tumors. J Nucl Med 51:669-673
35. Campana D, Ambrosini V, Pezzilli R et al (2010) Standardized uptake values of ^{68}Ga-DOTANOC PET: a promising prognostic tool in neuroendocrine tumors. J Nucl Med 51:353-359
36. Mankoff DA, Link JM, Linden HM et al (2008) Tumor receptor imaging. J Nucl Med 49:149S-163S
37. Haug A, Auernhammer CJ, Wängler B et al (2009) Intraindividual comparison of ^{68}Ga-DOTA-TATE and ^{18}F-DOPA PET in patients with well-differentiated metastatic neuroendocrine tumours. Eur J Nucl Med Mol Imaging 36:765-770
38. Mohnike K, Blankenstein O, Minn H et al (2008) ^{18}F-DOPA positron emission tomography for preoperative localization in congenital hyperinsulinism. Horm Res 70:65-72
39. Garin E, Le Jeune F, Devillers A et al (2009) Predictive value of ^{18}F-FDG PET and somatostatin receptor scintigraphy in patients with metastatic endocrine tumors. J Nucl Med 50:858-864
40. Mankoff DA, Eary JF, Link JM et al (2007) Tumor-specific positron emission tomography imaging in patients: ^{18}F-fluorodeoxyglucose and beyond. Clin Cancer Res 13:3460-3469
41. Lenders JW, Eisenhofer G, Mannelli M et al (2005) Phaeochromocytoma. Lancet 366:665-675
42. Kayani I, Bomanji JB, Groves A et al (2008) Functional imaging of neuroendocrine tumors with combined PET/CT using ^{68}Ga-DOTA-TATE (DOTA-DPhe^1,Tyr^3-octreotate) and ^{18}F-FDG. Cancer 112:2447-2455
43. Cremonesi M, Ferrari M, Bodei L et al (2006) Dosimetry in patients undergoing ^{177}Lu-DOTATATE therapy with indications for ^{90}Y-DOTATATE. Eur J Nucl Med Mol Imaging 33:S102
44. Cremonesi M, Ferrari M, Zoboli S et al (1999) Biokinetics and dosimetry in patients administered with ^{111}In-DOTA-Tyr^3-octreotide: implications for internal radiotherapy with ^{90}Y-DOTATOC. Eur J Nucl Med Mol Imaging 26:877-886
45. Kwekkeboom DJ, Teunissen JJ, Bakker WH et al (2005) Radiolabeled somatostatin analog ^{177}Lu-DOTA^0, Tyr^3-octreotate in patients with endocrine gastroenteropancreatic tumors. J Clin Oncol 23:2754-2762
46. Bernard BF, Krenning EP, Breeman WA et al (1997) D-lysine reduction of indium-111 octreotide and yttrium-90 octreotide renal uptake. J Nucl Med 38:1929-1933
47. Brans B, Bodei L, Giammarile F et al (2007) Clinical radionuclide therapy dosimetry: the quest for the "Holy Gray". Eur J Nucl Med Mol Imaging 34:772-786

48. de Jong M, Krenning EP (2002) New advances in peptide receptor radionuclide therapy. J Nucl Med 43:617-620
49. Valkema R, Pauwels SA, Kvols LK et al (2005) Long-term follow-up of renal function after peptide receptor radiation therapy with ^{90}Y-DOTA^0,Tyr^3-octreotide and ^{177}Lu-DOTA^0, Tyr^3-octreotate. J Nucl Med 46:83S-91S
50. Davi MV, Bodei L, Francia G et al (2006) Carcinoid crisis induced by receptor radionuclide therapy with ^{90}Y-DOTATOC in a case of liver metastases from bronchial neuroendocrine tumor (atypical carcinoid). J Endocrinol Invest 29:563-567
51. de Keizer B, van Aken MO, Feelders RA et al (2008) Hormonal crises following receptor radionuclide therapy with the radiolabeled somatostatin analogue ^{177}Lu-DOTA^0, Tyr^3-octreotate. Eur J Nucl Med Mol Imaging 35:749-755
52. Otte A, Herrmann R, Heppeler A et al (1999) Yttrium-90 DOTATOC: first clinical results. Eur J Nucl Med Mol Imaging 26:1439-1447
53. Waldherr C, Pless M, Maecke HR et al (2002) Tumor response and clinical benefit in neuroendocrine tumors after 7.4 GBq ^{90}Y-DOTATOC. J Nucl Med 43:610-616
54. Kwekkeboom DJ, Mueller-Brand J, Paganelli G et al (2005) Overview of results of peptide receptor radionuclide therapy with 3 radiolabeled somatostatin analogs. J Nucl Med 46:62S-66S

Targeted and Other Non-receptor-mediated Therapies

12

Sara Cingarlini, Chiara Trentin, Elisabetta Grego and Giampaolo Tortora

12.1 Introduction

Neuroendocrine neoplasms (NENs) are a relatively rare form of cancer whose incidence has sharply increased in the last decade. The diagnosis and treatment of these tumors have evolved in parallel. The recent 2010 WHO classification started a nosological (r)evolution based on a clearer distinction between: (1) neuroendocrine tumor and carcinoma and (2) grading and staging. Moreover, only a few months ago, the FDA approved everolimus and sunitinib for daily clinical use in patients with advanced "well/moderately" differentiated pancreatic NENs (PanNENs) [1].

National databases and data collected by referral centers have shown that gastro-entero-pancreatic (GEP)-NENs are most frequently located in the jejunum/ileum and pancreas, with a relative incidence of 16–29% and 31–34%, respectively. Moreover, they are characterized by higher loco-regional and distant metastatic spread; with an out-of-organ spread rate of 71–89% and 54–86%, respectively, making them the predominant NENs in oncological/non-surgical series [2].

In addition to the biological heterogeneity of NENs, the rarity of the disease and the paucity of related series have been problematic for the quality of clinical trials, such that interpretation of the results is often challenging. A recent survey of studies published between 2000 and 2010 reported six phase III and 34 phase II trials, the majority of which (78%) were single-arm studies, often including more than one tumor type (43%). Furthermore, tumor differentiation and Ki67 index were reported in only 37% and 12% of the ana-

G. Tortora (✉)
Department of Medical Oncology, "G.B. Rossi" University Hospital,
Verona, Italy
e-mail: giampaolo.tortora@univr.it

P. Pederzoli and C. Bassi (eds.), *Uncommon Pancreatic Neoplasms*,
Updates in Surgery
DOI: 10.1007/978-88-470-2673-5_12, © Springer-Verlag Italia 2013

135

lyzed trials, respectively [3]. As a further methodological drawback, the results of these studies were frequently ambiguous, due to the lack of routine evaluation of disease status at the time of enrollment. In the largest published series of NENs/carcinomas (NEN/Cs) treated with ^{177}Lu-DOTA-TATE, only 43% of patients had documented progressive disease (PD) before peptide receptor radionuclide therapy (PRRT) enrollment [4]. Not even in the PRO-MID study, which evaluated the ability of somatostatin analogues (SSAs) to control the growth of advanced midgut well-differentiated NENs, was PD a required inclusion or stratification criterion. Disease status was reported in only 50% of the published trials and only 20% of them included progressive cases at baseline [5].

Unlike patients with other types of cancers, those with NENs can benefit from a multi-disciplinary approach, including in the metastatic setting. Strategies including surgery for loco-regional or metastatic disease, even if only for tumor debulking purposes, have been proven to confer a survival advantage in some patients. Based on a SEER retrospective survival analysis of 728 patients with PanNENs, surgery for locally advanced and metastatic disease is advocated in selected cases due to the significant survival advantage: 129 vs. 64 months for resected vs. non-resected localized metastatic disease, and 60 vs. 31 months for distant metastatic disease [6]. In addition to aggressive approaches to the management of advanced NENs, nowadays the primary need is to determine sequential strategies that optimize the use of all therapeutic options. Randomized head-to-head trials comparing different therapeutic strategies are lacking, while indirect and retrospective comparisons of published data are potentially misleading.

Another highly current topic is the effectiveness of response evaluation in patients receiving the new medical therapeutic options. While the efficacy of chemotherapeutic regimens can, in most cases, be properly assessed according to WHO or RECIST parameters, the molecular targeted agents require different criteria, as tumor size measurements according to RECIST could underestimate the real clinical benefit of these tailored drugs. Perfusion/functional computed tomography (CT), contrast-enhanced magnetic resonance imaging (MRI), and positron emission tomography (PET) with 2-[fluorine-18]-fluoro-2-deoxy-D-glucose (FDG) are emerging as novel resources for dimensional and/or functional imaging of these tumors. Although still limited in numbers, the experiences described to date with perfusional CT scans are encouraging. In 22 patients with advanced carcinoid tumors and liver metastases, bevacizumab treatment significantly reduced tumor blood flow and volume compared to baseline and to the untreated controls. However, due to the limited number of patients, a significant correlation with standard outcome parameters could not be determined [7]. In a larger series of patients with advanced low-to intermediate-grade NENs, the combination of bevacizumab and everolimus resulted in a partial remission (PR) rate of 26%. A functional CT (fCT) evaluation showed a significant association between standard RECIST criteria and fCT parameters (baseline permeability surface, blood flow mean transit time, intralesional blood flow and volume) in responding patients [8].

Clearly, these novel therapeutic approaches demand a new analytical approach, one that integrates a wide range of clinical and imaging skills, resources and perspectives in disease evaluation and the development of unambiguous guidelines regarding the treatment of these patients.

12.2 Chemotherapy

In contrast to the low chemosensitivity of other NENs, PanNENs show moderate/good responsiveness to some antiblastic agents. In a literature search of publications since 1980, we collected 35 papers (published in extenso) and nine abstracts addressing the issue of chemotherapy for PanNENs. Among the papers, 14 were retrospective surveys (mono- or poly-centric) and 21 were prospective studies (of which only three were randomized). Ten were "PanNEN-dedicated" and ten others were selected because they included at least ten cases of PanNENs; seven studies also enrolled patients with poorly differentiated disease. Mono- and poly-chemotherapy were evaluated in six and 16 trials, respectively, either as a single-arm study or in the context of a randomized trial. Regarding progressive disease, in three of the 20 studies (15%) it was among the inclusion criteria, while in six of the 20 (30%) it specifically was not. In the remaining studies, no such information was provided. The great majority of enrolled patients had undergone previous treatment, most of them with an SSA.

Single-agent chemotherapy in PanNEN was shown to have a limited role. Dacarbazin (DTIC) yielded a response rate (RR) of 26%, with a median progression-free survival (PFS) of 10 months [9]; for streptozototcin (STZ), the RR was 21–36% with a PFS of 16.5–33 months [10, 11], and with chlorzotocin (CTZ) a PR of 30% with a PFS of 17 months was reported [12]. Temozolomide was tested in a heterogeneous population of 36 patients with thoraco-abdominal NENs, including only 12 PanNENs; the global RR was 8% and PFS did not exceed 7 months [13].

In one of the first random controlled trials (RCTs) comparing mono- and poly-chemotherapy in the setting of PanNENs, STZ was tested against the combination of STZ and 5-fluorouracil (STZ/5-FU); both the RR of 36 vs. 63% and the overall survival (OS) of 16.5 vs. 26 months significantly favored the combination arm. The same study compared, in a three-arm RCT, CTZ alone, and two STZ-based regimens: STZ/5-FU and doxorubicin/STZ (ADM/STZ); the latter was significantly superior to STZ/5-FU in terms of RR, PFS, and OS (45 vs. 69%, 13 vs. 22 months, and 17 vs. 26 months, respectively) [12]. The same combination was not able to reproduce similar results in two other poly-chemotherapy single-arm retrospective studies, in which STZ/ADM resulted in a RR of 6–36%, a median PFS of 3.9–16 months, and an OS of 20.2–24 months [14-17]. Oxaliplatin, which has a moderate activity in well-/intermediate-differentiated NENs, was tested together with capecitabine in a series of 40 patients with WD-NEN (well-differentiated neuroendocrine neoplasm) (15 PanNENs); a PR was obtained in 27% of the patients, with a median PFS of 20 months and an OS of 40 months [18]. However, when used in combination with gemcitabine, oxaliplatin did not have a similar efficacy, probably because of the limited activity of gemcitabine in this histotype [19]. The GEMOX regimen was tested in a heterogeneous group of 20 patients with thoracic, GEP, and unknown-primary NENs; (only 5 PanNENs). The overall RR was 17%, with a median PFS of only 7 months and an OS of 23.4 months [20].

Intensification with three-drug regimens has produced only a slight increase in efficacy. The attempt to intensify regimens by adding a third drug to the above-mentioned doublets, although never tested in a RCT, does not seem to lead to significant clinical improvement. Dacarbazin and cisplatinum were the most frequently tested drugs in combination with STZ/5-FU or 5-FU/ADM backbones. The RR for the triplets ranged from 19.5% to 58%; the PFS from 9.1 to 21 months, and the OS from 21 to 38 months [21-25].

The combination of temozolomide and capecitabine has shown promising results. The efficacy of this regimen was tested in 30 patients with PanNENs, yielding a PR of 70%, a median PFS of 18 months, and an OS of 92% at 2 years [26]. The encouraging activity of this doublet has a biological rationale; the DNA repair enzyme O6-methylguanine DNA methyltransferase (MGMT) contributes to the resistance of tumor cells to temozolomide. As demonstrated by a recent immunohistochemistry analysis of NEN samples, 51% and 0% of pancreatic and small-intestine NENs, respectively, showed MGMT deficiency [27]. This could represent the biological basis for the higher sensitivity of pancreatic, compared to other NENs following temozolomide treatment. Whether MGMT deficiency can serve as a predictive marker of response to temozolomide warrants further studies. Similarly, the intracellular depletion of MGMT by the co-administration of capecitabine may account for the observed synergistic effect.

The most relevant features of the main chemotherapy trials are summarized in Table 12.1.

12.3   Targeted Therapies

The PI3K-Akt-mTOR pathway is a key regulator pathway in the biology of NENs [28-35] and its constitutive activation has been described in many malignancies, including these tumors. Some genetic syndromes have evidenced the role of a loss or the down-regulation of tumor suppressor phosphatase and tensin homologue (PTEN) or tuberous sclerosis 2 (TSC-2) in the constitutive activation of the PI3K-Akt-mTOR pathway. These alterations have been frequently described also in NEN tumorigenesis; 85% of PanNENs show altered levels of TSC2 and/or PTEN and in both cases the degree of down-regulation inversely correlates with prognosis, as demonstrated in a

Table 12.1 Main clinical studies with chemotherapy

Author (year)	CT (mono-CT)	Type	Total pts n°	n° PanNETs	PFS (months)	OS (months)	RR (%)
Brizzi et al. (2009) [42]	5FU (+Octreotide LAR)	NEN	29	13	22.6	NR	24.1
Ekeblad et al. (2007) [13]	TMZ	NEN	36	12	7	16	8
Ramanhatan et al. (2001) [9]	DTIC	NEN	50	50	10	19.3	26
Moertel et al. (1992) [43]	CZT	NEN	105	33	17	18	NA
Moertel et al. (1980) [10]	STZ	NEN	52	52	33	42	21
Broder et al. (1973) [11]	STZ	NEN	84	42	NA	16.5	36
CT (doublets)							
Strosberg et al. (2011) [26]	CPT/TMZ	NEN	30	30	18	NA	70
Bajetta et al. (2007) [18]	XELOX	NEN/NEC	40	15	20	40	27
McCollum et al. (2004) [14]	STZ/DOXO	NEN	16	16	3.9	20.2	6
Delaunoit et al. (2004) [15]	DOXO/STZ	NEN	45	45	16	24	36
Fjallskog et al. (2001) [44]	CDDP/VP16	NEN/NEC	36	15	9	NA	36
Mitry et al. (1999) [45]	CDDP/VP16	NEN	12	4	2.3	17.6	9.1
Cheng et al. (1999) [17]	STZ/5FU	NEN	16	16	NA	NR	6
Moertel et al. (1992) [43]	5FU/STZ	NEN	105	34	13	17	NA
Moertel et al. (1992) [43]	DOXO/STZ	NEN	105	38	22	26	NA
Moertel et al. (1991) [46]	CDDP/VP16	NEN	45	14	4	15.5	14
Eriksson et al. (1990) [16]	STZ/DOXO	NEN	59	25	27.5	NA	NA
CT (triplets)							
Turner et al. (2010) [21]	STZ/5FU/CDDP	NEN/NEC	82	49	9.1	31.5	38.2
Walter et al. (2010) [22]	5FU/DCZ/EPI	NEN	39	16	17	27	58
Kouvaraki et al. (2004) [23]	5FU/DOXO/STZ	NEN	84	84	18	37	39
Bajetta et al. (2002) [24]	DCZ/5FU/EPI	NEN	82	28	21	38	19.5
Rivera E et al. (1998) [25]	STZ/DOXO/5 FU	NEN	12	12	15	21	54.5

series of 72 patients with PanNENs [36]. Furthermore genome sequencing together with expression profiling has identified somatic mutations implicated in the self-maintenance of activated signaling along this pathway.

Data from clinical trials have supported the central role of the PI3K-Akt-mTOR pathway in PanNEN tumorigenesis. In the RADIANT-1 study, everolimus was administered either alone or in combination with octreotide long-acting release (LAR), if such treatment was ongoing at baseline. The primary endpoint was RR in the largest stratum of everolimus monotherapy (n = 115 patients). In these patients, the RR was 9.6% vs. 4.4% for patients in the everolimus + octreotide stratum. No conclusions could be drawn regarding possible interactions between everolimus and SSA because: (a) it was not a randomized study; (b) the number of patients in the everolimus stratum greatly exceeded that in the combination arm; and (c) the biology of the patients enrolled in the two strata differed. Specifically, in the stratum with everolimus alone, 19% of SSA-naïve patients had a syndromic tumor, including those who might have benefited from inclusion in the stratum with everolimus and SSA. PFS in the SSA + everolimus stratum was longer than in the everolimus alone stratum (16.7 vs. 9.7 months) [37]. The antitumor activity and safety of everolimus in the treatment of NENs confirmed the conclusion of a previous phase II study. This trial similarly intended to evaluate the activity of everolimus in combination with octreotide LAR in patients with advanced PanNEN. The overall RR (ORR) was somewhat higher than in RADIANT-1 (30% in the arm comprising patients treated with the same everolimus dose). However, the population differed between the studies: in the first study, the percentage of patients (34%) enrolled with stable disease was higher and a minority of them (43%) were pretreated with chemotherapy [38].

The RADIANT-3 study further explored the role of everolimus in the management of 410 patients with advanced PanNENs, in a randomized fashion against placebo. Pretreatment with chemotherapy was a stratification criteria and SSA treatment was allowed in both arms during the trial. The trial design enabled cross-over at PD, with PFS as the only suitable primary endpoint in order to evaluate clinical benefit. PR, defined according to RECIST, was obtained in 5% of the patients in the everolimus arm but 64% of patients receiving the drug experienced some degree of tumor shrinkage, compared to 21% in the placebo arm. In addition, everolimus reduced tumor proliferation, as shown by a decreased in the Ki67 index on paired re-biopsies. However, the most striking benefit following everolimus treatment was longer time to disease progression. Specifically, the adjudicated central review PFS was 11.4 and 5.4 months for the everolimus and placebo arms, respectively, resulting in a reduction of the risk of progression for the experimental arm of nearly 65%. No subgroup was disadvantaged: neither chemotherapy-pretreated patients nor those with moderately differentiated tumors. The homogeneous selection of patients with PanNENs and progressive disease together with the adequate sample size enrolled renders the results of this trial essentially unquestionable. Nonetheless, some concerns remain regarding the biology of the tumors included in the study, since: (a) 70% of the patients had a diagnosis of PD within 3 months before enrollment and nothing is known about pre-progression disease behavior; (b) 17% of the patients had moderately differentiated tumors for which not even a median Ki67 was reported [39]. The lack of this information could make it difficult to compare this trial with others. The RR and PFS obtained with everolimus of 5% and 11.4 months, respectively, must be compared with those obtained with other strategies. PRRT with Lu-DOTA-octreotate on Octreoscan-positive PanNENs lead to RRs ranging from 36% for non-functioning pancreatic tumors to 60% for insulinomas, with a global PFS of nearly 40 months. STZ-based chemotherapy, according to a historical study, obtained an RR in 69% of PanNEN-bearing patients, with a median PFS of 22 months. Head-to-head comparisons, in the context of a phase III RCT, of the currently available therapeutic strategies are warranted.

NENs are highly vascularized tumors. High levels of VEGF expression by PanNENs is a negative prognostic factor related to higher microvessel density, a higher incidence of metastases, and a shorter PFS. Many different anti-angiogenic drugs are now available for clinical use, both as specific target agents or as pleiotropic kinase inhibitors. Bevacizumab was tested in a phase II randomized study against pegylated interferon-α (PEG-IFNα) in a population of 44 patients with carcinoids (excluding pancreas primaries) who received a stable dose of octreotide. In the bevacizumab arm, 18% of patients achieved a PR, with 77% SD in contrast to the PEG-IFNα arm, in which no PR was documented and SD was obtained in 68% of patients [8]. The results of many trials, including bevacizumab in combination with either chemotherapy or other targeted agents, in patients with advanced, are awaited. A prospective randomized phase III trial testing bevacizumab + octreotide LAR vs. IFNα + octreotide LAR, as well as other phase II single-arm clinical studies (TMZ + bevacizumab, CAPOX + bevacizumab, FOLFOX + bevacizumab, everolimus + bevacizumab) are ongoing.

Sunitinib was also tested as anti-angiogenetic multi-target agent in NENs. The first experience, in a single-arm phase II trial, showed promising results. In that study, 109 patients with advanced NENs (66 PanNENs and 41 carcinoids) were evaluated. A PR was obtained in 16.7% of the PanNEN patients, with a median PFS of 7.7 months; among those with carcinoids, the RR was 2.4%, with a PFS of 10.2 months [40]. The assumed major clinical benefit of sunitinib in the subgroup of patients with PanNENs led to a phase III study in which only patients with advanced PanNENs were enrolled. The 171 patients were randomly assigned to receive sunitinib (37.5 mg/day) or placebo together with best supportive care. Patients with PD in the placebo arm were allowed to enter an open-label sunitinib extension protocol; thus, the primary end point was necessarily PFS, as in the everolimus registrative phase III study. Noteworthy baseline characteristics of the enrolled patients were: 22% with tumors having a Ki67 > 10% and 66% pretreated with chemotherapy in the experimental arm. Patients in both arms were allowed to receive SSAs according to the investigators' discretion. Both these percentages were well-balanced in the placebo arm. After assessment of the data on 154 patients, the safety monitoring committee recommended discontinuation of the trial because of the large number of deaths and serious adverse events in the placebo group. At that time point, a RR of 9.3% and 0% were recorded in the experimental and placebo arms, respectively. A statistically significant difference in PFS between the two arms was also determined (11.4 vs. 5.5 months). Both subgroups of patients benefited from sunitinib but the hazard ratio for progression in the experimental arm compared to placebo seemed to favor patients with a Ki67 index ≤5 % [41].

The most relevant features of the main trials with target agents are summarized in Table 12.2.

Table 12.2 Main clinical studies with targeted agents

Author (year)	Therapy	Type	Total pts (n)	Pan NENs (n)	PFS (months)	OS (months)	RR (%)
Yao et al. (2011) [39]	Everolimus	NEN	410	207	11	NR	5
Yao et al. (2010) [37]	Everolimus	NEN	160	115	9.7	24,9	9.6
Pavel et al. (2011) [47]	Everolimus + Oct LAR	NEN	216	5	16.4	NA	NA
Yao et al. (2008) [8]	Everolimus 5/10 + Oct LAR	NEN	30	29	12.5	NR	13
Duran et al. (2006) [48]	Temsirolimus	NEN	37	15	10.6	NR (86.5%) at 2 ys	6.7
Raymond et al. (2011) [41]	Sunitinib	NEN	171	86	11.4	NA	7
Deeks et al. (2011) [49]	Sunitinib	NEN	86	86	12.6	30,5	9.3
Barriuso et al. (2010) [50]	Sunitinib	NEN	40	28	12	NR	7
Kulke et al. (2008) [40]	Sunitinib	NEN	109	66	10.5	NA (83.4%) at 2 ys	17 / 17
Castellano et al. (2010) [52]	Sorafenib + Beva	NEN	44	13	10	NA	16.7
Yao et al. (2008) [8]	Oct LAR + Beva /IFN PEG	NEN	44	0	16.5	NA	NA
Hobday et al. (2007) [53]	Sorafenib	NEN	93	43	NA	NA	7.5
Kulke et al. (2006) [54]	Temozolamide + Beva	NEN	34	18	NA	NA	NA

NA, Not assessed; *NR*, not reached; *NEN*, neuroendocrine neoplasm.

Recent developments in the setting of NENs underline some of the most rapidly evolving areas in the oncologic panorama. Although univocal and shared treatment strategies have yet to be defined, the growing number of currently available drugs holds promise as the basis of a firmer and more successful therapeutic future.

References

1. Klimstra DS, Modlin IR, Coppola D et al (2010) The pathologic classification of neuroendocrine tumors: a review of nomenclature, grading, and staging systems. Pancreas 39:707-712
2. Yao JC, Hassan M, Phan A et al (2008) One hundred years after "carcinoid": epidemiology of and prognostic factors for neuroendocrine tumors in 35,825 cases in the United States. J Clin Oncol 26:3063-3072
3. Walter T, Krzyzanowska MK (2012) Quality of clinical trials Gastro-Entero-Pancreatic Neuroendocrine Tumors. Neuroendocrinology [Epub ahead of print]
4. Kwekkeboom DJ, de Herder WW, Kam BL et al (2008) Treatment with the radiolabeled somatostatin analog [177 Lu-DOTA 0,Tyr3] octreotate: toxicity, efficacy, and survival. J Clin Oncol 26:2124-2130
5. Rinke A, Muller HH, Schade-Brittinger C et al (2009) Placebo-controlled, double-blind, prospective, randomized study on the effect of octreotide LAR in the controltumor growth in patients with metastatic neuroendocrine midgut tumors: a report from the PROMID Study Group. J Clin Oncol 27:4656-4663
6. Hill JS, McPhee JT, McDade TP et al (2009) Pancreatic neuroendocrine tumors: the impact of surgical resection on survival. Cancer 115:741-751
7. Yao JC, Phan AT, Fogleman D et al (2010) Randomized run-in study of bevacizumab (B) and everolimus (E) in low- to intermediate-grade neuroendocrine tumors (LGNETs) using perfusion CT as functional biomarker. Journal of Clinical Oncology. ASCO Annual Meeting Proceedings (Post-Meeting Edition) 28 (15 suppl): 4002
8. Yao JC, Phan A, Hoff PM et al (2008) Targeting vascular endothelial growth factor in advanced carcinoid tumor: a random assignment phase II study of depot octreotide with bevacizumab and pegylated interferon alpha-2b. J Clin Oncol 26:1316-1323
9. Ramanathan RK, Cnaan RK, Carbone PP, Hailed DG (2001) Original article Phase II trial of dacarbazine (DTIC) in advanced pancreatic islet cell carcinoma . Study of the Eastern Cooperative Oncology Group-E6282. Annals of Oncology 12:1139-1143
10. Moertel CG, Hanley JA, Johnson LA (1980) Streptozocin alone compared with streptozocin plus fluorouracil in the treatment of advanced islet-cell carcinoma. N Engl J Med 303:1189-1194
11. Broder LE, Carter SK (1973) Pancreatic islet cell carcinoma. I. Clinical features of 52 patients. Annals of internal medicine 79:101-107
12. Moertel CG, Lefkopoulo M, Lipsitz S et al (1992) Streptozocin-doxorubicin, streptozocin-fluorouracil or chlorozotocin in the treatment of advanced islet-cell carcinoma. N Engl J Med 326:519-523
13. Ekeblad S, Sundin A, Janson ET et al (2007) Temozolomide as monotherapy is effective in treatment of advanced malignant neuroendocrine tumors. Clin Cancer Res 13:2986-2991
14. McCollum D, Kulke MH, Ryan DP et al (2004) Lack of Efficacy of Streptozocin and Doxorubicin in Patients With Advanced Pancreatic Endocrine Tumors. Am J Clin Oncol 27:485-488
15. Delaunoit T, Ducreux M, Boige V et al (2004) The doxorubicin-streptozotocin combination for the treatment of advanced well-differentiated pancreatic endocrine carcinoma; a judicious option? Eur J Cancer 40:515-520

16. Eriksson B, Skogseid B, Lundqvist G et al (1990) Medical treatment and long-term survival in a prospective study of 84 patients with endocrine pancreatic tumors. Cancer 65:1883-1890
17. Cheng PN, Saltz LB (1999) Failure to confirm major objective antitumor activity for streptozocin and doxorubicin in the treatment of patients with advanced islet cell carcinoma. Cancer 86:944-948
18. Bajetta E, Catena L, Procopio G et al (2007) Are capecitabine and oxaliplatin (XELOX) suitable treatments for progressing low-grade and high-grade neuroendocrine tumours? Cancer Chemother Pharmacol 59:637-642
19. Kulke MH, Kim H, Clark JW et al (2004) A Phase II trial of gemcitabine for metastatic neuroendocrine tumors. Cancer 101:934-939
20. Cassier P, Walter T, Eymard B et al (2009) Gemcitabine and oxaliplatin combination chemotherapy for metastatic well-differentiated neuroendocrine carcinomas: a single-center experience. Cancer 115:3392-3399
21. Turner NC, Strauss SJ, Sarker D et al (2010) Chemotherapy with 5-fluorouracil, cisplatin and streptozocin for neuroendocrine tumours. Br J Cancer 102:1106-1112
22. Walter T, Bruneton D, Cassier PA et al (2010) Evaluation of the combination 5-fluorouracil, dacarbazine, and epirubicin in patients with advanced well-differentiated neuroendocrine tumors. Clin Colorectal Cancer 9:248-254
23. Kouvaraki M, Ajani JA, Hoff P et al (2004). Fluorouracil, doxorubicin, and streptozocin in the treatment of patients with locally advanced and metastatic pancreatic endocrine carcinomas. J Clin Oncol 22:4762-4771
24. Bajetta E, Ferrari L, Procopio G et al (2002) Efficacy of a chemotherapy combination for the treatment of metastatic neuroendocrine tumours. Ann Oncol 13:614-621
25. Rivera E, Ajani JA (1998) Doxoribicin, streptozocin, and 5-fluorouracil chemotherapy for patients with metastaticislet-cell carcinoma. Am J Clin Oncol 21:36-38
26. Strosberg JR, Fine RL,Choi J et al (2011) First-line chemotherapy with capecitabine and temozolomide in patients with metastatic pancreatic endocrine carcinomas. Cancer 117:268-275
27. Kulke MH, Hornick JL, Frauenhoffer C et al (2009) O6-methylguanine DNA methyltransferase deficiency and response to temozolomide-based therapy in patients with neuroendocrine tumors. Clin Res Cancer Res 15:338-345
28. Chiu CW, Nozawa H, Hanahan D (2010) Survival Benefit With Proapoptotic Molecular and Pathologic Responses From Dual Targeting of Mammalian Target of Rapamycin and Epidermal Growth Factor Receptor in a Preclinical Model of Pancreatic Neuroendocrine Carcinogenesis. Clinical Oncology 28:4425-4433
29. Di Florio, Adesso L, Pedrotti S et al (2011) Src kinase activity coordinates cell adhesion and spreading with activation of mammalian target of rapamycin in pancreatic endocrine tumour cells. Endocr Relat Cancer 18:541-554
30. Couderc C, Poncet G, Villaume K et al (2011) Targeting the PI3K / mTOR Pathway in Murine Endocrine Cell Lines In Vitro and in Vivo Effects on Tumor Cell Growth. Am J Pathol 178:336-344
31. Jiao Y, Shi C, Edil BH (2011) DAXX/A, MEN1, AND Mtor pathway genes are frequently altered in pancreatic neuroendocrin tumors. Science 331:1199-1203
32. Kasajima A, Pavel M, Darb-Esfahani S et al (2011) mTOR expression and activity patterns in gastroenteropancreatic neuroendocrine tumours. Endocrine-Related Cancer 18:181-192
33. Righi L, Volante M, Rapa I et al (2010) Meammalian target of rapamycin signaling activation patterns in neuroendocrine tumors of the lung. Endocrine-Related Cancer 17:977-987
34. Zatelli MC, Minoia M, Martini C et al (2010) Everolimus as a new potential antiproliferative agent in aggressive human bronchial carcinoids. Endocrine-Related Cancer 17:719-729
35. Shida T, Kichimoto T, Furuia M et al (2010) Expression of an activated mammalian target of rapamycin (mTOR) in gastroenteropancreatic neuroendocrine tumors. Cancer Chemoter Pharmacol 65:889-893
36. Missiaglia E, Dalai I, Barbi S et al (2010) Pancreatic endocrine tumors: expression profiling evidences a role for AKT-mTOR pathway. J Clin Oncol 28:245-255

12 Targeted and Other Non-receptor-mediated Therapies

37. Yao JC, Lombard-Bohas C, Baudin E et al (2010) Daily oral everolimus activity in patients with metastatic pancreatic neuroendocrine tumors after failure of cytotoxic chemotherapy: a phase II trial. J Clin Oncol 28:69-76
38. Yao JC, Phan AT, Chang DZ et al (2008) Efficacy of RAD001 (everolimus) and octreotide LAR in advanced low- to intermediate-grade neuroendocrine tumors: results of a phase II study. J Clin Oncol 26:4311-4318
39. Yao JC, Shah MH, Ito T et al (2011) Everolimus for Advanced Pancreatic Neuroendocrine Tumors. N Engl J Med 364:514-523
40. Kulke MH, Lenz HJ, Meropol NJ et al (2008) Activity of sunitinib in patients with advanced neuroendocrine tumors. J Clin Oncol 26:3403-3410
41. Raymond E, Danan L, Raul Jl et al (2011) Sunitinib malate for the treatment of pancreatic neuroendocrine tumors. N Engl J Med 364:501-513
42. Brizzi M, Berruti A, Ferrero A (2009) Continuous 5-fluorouracil infusion plus long acting octreotide in advanced well-differentiated neuroendocrine carcinomas. A phase II trial of the Piemonte Oncology Network. BMC Cancer 9:1-8
43. Moertel CG, Lefkopoulo M, Lipsitz S et al (1992) Streptozocin-doxorubicin, streptozocin-fluorouracil or chlorozotocin in the treatment of advanced islet-cell carcinoma. N Engl J Med 326:519-523
44. Fjällskog ML, Granberg DP, Welin SL et al (2001) Treatment with cisplatin and etoposide in patients with neuroendocrine tumors. Cancer 92:1101-1107
45. Mitry E, Baudin E, Ducreux M et al (1999) Treatment of poorly differentiated neuroendocrine tumours with etoposide and cisplatin. Br J Cancer 81:1351-1355
46. Moertel CG, Kvols LK, O'Connell MJ et al (1991) Treatment of neuroendocrine carcinomas with combined etoposide and cisplatin. Evidence of major therapeutic activity in the anaplastic variants of these neoplasms. Cancer 68: 227-232
47. Pavel ME, Hainsworth JD, Baudin E et al (2011) Everolimus plus octreotide long-acting repeatable for the treatment of advanced neuroendocrine tumours associated with carcinoid syndrome (RADIANT-2): a randomised, placebo-controlled, phase 3 study. Lancet 378:2005-2012
48. Duran I, Kortmansky J, Singh D et al (2006) A phase II clinical and pharmacodynamic study of temsirolimus in advanced neuroendocrine carcinomas. Br J Cancer 95:1148-1154
49. Deeks ED, Raymond E (2011) Sunitinib: in advanced, well differentiated pancreatic neuroendocrine tumors. Bio Drugs 25:307-316
50. Barriuso J, Grande E, Quindós Varela M et al (2010) Sunitinib efficacy and tolerability in patients with neuroendocrine tumors out of a trial: a spanish multicenter cohort. Annals of Oncology 21 (Supplement 8):847P
51. Kulke MH, Lenz HJ, Meropol NJ et al (2008) Activity of Sunitinib in Patients With Advanced. Neuroendocrine Tumors. J Clin Oncol 26:3403-3410
52. Castellano D, Capdevilla J, Salazar R et al (2010) Sorafenib and bevacizumab combination targeted therapy in advanced neuroendocrine tumor: a phase ii study of spanish neuroendocrine tumor group (getne-0801). Annals of Oncology 21 (Suppl 8):850P
53. Hobday TJ, Rubin J, Holen K et al (2007) MC044h, a phase II trial of sorafenib in patients (pts) with metastatic neuroendocrine tumors (NET): A Phase II Consortium (P2C) study. Journal of Clinical Oncology, 2007 ASCO Annual Meeting Proceedings (Post-Meeting Edition). 25 (20 Suppl):4504
54. Kulke MH, Stuart K, Earle CC et al (2006) A phase II study of temozolomide and bevacizumab in patients with advanced neuroendocrine tumors. J Clin Oncol, ASCO Annual Meeting Proceedings 24 (20 Suppl): 4044

Part III

Uncommon Pancreatic Solid Neoplasms

Giovanni Butturini

Historically, pancreatic tumor was synonymous with pancreatic ductal adenocarcinoma, the histotype accounting for the vast majority of all pancreatic neoplasms. Nowadays, ductal adenocarcinoma still represents the most frequent neoplasm and almost universally an invincible disease, with a very poor prognosis for these patients. However, during the last two decades, other histotypes have been described that have gained considerable interest due to their unique histopathological characteristics, specific genetic alterations, and natural history.

Besides neuroendocrine and cystic tumors of the pancreas, which represent the opposite end in the spectrum of pancreatic tumors and are extensively discussed elsewhere in this book, in this section we describe a miscellany of diseases, ranging from solid masses mimicking pancreatic cancer to rare primary or secondary tumors located in the pancreas, often identified only after surgical excision. Differentiating between these rare histotypes and ductal adenocarcinoma and other well-known neoplasms, such as cystic and neuroendocrine tumors, is of paramount importance, as both adjuvant treatment and prognosis may be different.

Thus, the aim of this section is to familiarize readers with the clinicopathological features, molecular biology, and radiological characteristics of uncommon pancreatic lesions. Furthermore, our recommendations for the diagnosis and clinical management of these rare conditions are outlined.

G. Butturini (✉)
Department of Surgery and Oncology, General Surgery Unit, Pancreas Center,
"G.B. Rossi" University Hospital,
Verona, Italy
e-mail: giovanni.butturini@ospedaleuniverona.it

P. Pederzoli and C. Bassi (eds.), *Uncommon Pancreatic Neoplasms,*
Updates in Surgery
DOI: 10.1007/978-88-470-2673-5_13, © Springer-Verlag Italia 2013

Rare Variants of Ductal Adenocarcinoma of the Pancreas

13

Paolo Regi, Marco Dal Molin, Federica Pedica,
Paola Capelli, Mirko D'Onofrio and Giovanni Butturini

Histologic variants of ductal adenocarcinoma are neoplasms characterized by a specific histological pattern different from that of conventional pancreatic cancer, which is typically an adenocarcinoma. It has been estimated that these variants account for 2–10% of all pancreatic ductal cancers.

13.1 Adenosquamous Carcinoma

Among rare pancreatic neoplasms, adenosquamous carcinoma (ASC) comprise 0.9–4.4% of all pancreatic malignancies [1-3]. These patients have a worse prognosis than those with the more common ductal pancreatic cancer. Little is known about this rare subtype, as its biological behavior has been derived only from case reports and small retrospective series, often with in homogeneous results that are, accordingly, difficult to compare. More recent reports have shown that the median survival rate of patients with ASC undergoing surgical resection with radical intent (R0-R1) along with adjuvant treatment (chemotherapy alone or in conjunction with external beam radiation) is similar to that of patients with resectable pancreatic cancer (PC) [4, 5].

13.1.1 Pathology and Genetics

The first histological description of ASC reported in the literature was that of Herxheimer, in 1907, who defined this unusual entity as "cancroide" [6]. The characteristic cellular mixture of squamous and adenomatous cellular lines led

---

P. Regi (✉)
Surgery Unit, Casa di cura "Dr. P. Pederzoli",
Peschiera del Garda (VR), Italy"
e-mail: paoloregi@tiscali.it

P. Pederzoli and C. Bassi (eds.), *Uncommon Pancreatic Neoplasms*,
Updates in Surgery
DOI: 10.1007/978-88-470-2673-5_13, © Springer-Verlag Italia 2013

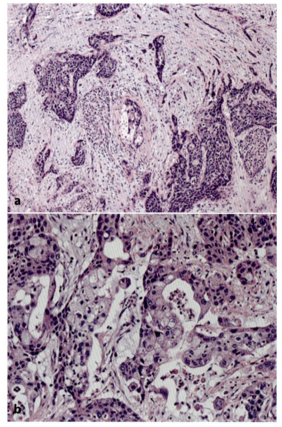

Fig. 13.1 a Squamous adenocarcinoma without keratinization. b Carcinoma with evident mucin secretion at seen at higher magnification

other authors to various definitions of ASC, such as adenoacanthoma, mixed squamous and adenocarcinoma, or mucoepidermoid carcinoma [2, 3].

It was not until 2000 that the World Health Organization clearly indicated the presence of at least 30% squamous cell carcinoma differentiation as a mandatory criterion for the diagnosis of ASC (Fig. 13.1). Since then, tumors showing a lower squamous proportion are designated as PC with "squamous differentiation" [7].

Many theories have been proposed to explain the origin of ASC. In the "squamous metaplasia theory," squamous metaplasia was postulated to occur as a result of ductal inflammation due to chronic pancreatitis or obstruction by an adenocarcinomatous tumor that ultimately became a malignant adenosquamous pancreatic tumor. A second theory, termed "the collision theory," suggested that two histologically distinct tumors, adenocarcinoma and squamous cell carcinoma, arise independently from different sites and then fuse. According to the third theory, the "differentiation theory," ASC reflects the

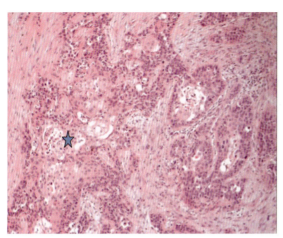

Fig. 13.2 Squamous cell carcinoma with aspects of squamous differentiation (*star*)

malignant differentiation of a pluripotent ductal cell into two distinct histological types.

Currently, the most widely accepted theory postulates a metaplasia from a focal adenocarcinomatous cancer towards a squamous histotype [2, 8, 9] (Fig. 13.2). This consideration originates from a common observation during specimen examination, i.e., that only adenocarcinomatous foci show a characteristic cytological spectrum from ductal hyperplasia to carcinoma in situ, and are typically surrounded by squamous cell lines without a transitional margin [8, 9]. Furthermore, even ASC with a particular squamous predominance consistently contains *KRAS2* gene mutations, similarly to the more common PC [8, 10-13].

13.1.2 Clinical Presentation and Diagnostic Work-up

The preoperative differential diagnosis between ASC and PC is often difficult. Similar to PC, ASC shows a slightly greater prevalence in males (M/F ratio: 1.5:1), with a mean age of 62 years. The most frequent symptoms at the time of presentation are weight loss, jaundice, and non-specific abdominal pain. Even the radiological and macroscopic appearance of ASC may completely mimic a typical PC [3, 8]. However, expression of the tumor markers CEA and CA 19-9 directly correlate with a more aggressive biological behavior and an advanced stage of disease [3, 8, 11, 14, 15].

Preoperatively, fine-needle aspiration (FNA) is a useful tool to obtain the correct diagnosis, although it requires careful pathological examination of the specimen in order to accurately distinguish the squamous cell cancer component from "atypical cells" (also referred to as "epidermoid"). The latter are also found in patients with chronic pancreatitis or in those undergoing endoscopic biliary stent placement [16, 17].

13.1.3 Clinical Management

By the time symptoms occur, the vast majority of patients with ASC will present with advanced disease and thus succumb early, due to local or systemic dissemination. A potentially curative surgical resection (R0-R1) of the tumor, followed by adjuvant treatment (chemoradiation) is the only therapeutic option that can potentially lead to a significantly better survival [5, 8, 11].

Indeed, in a recent retrospective study by Voong et al. [5], based on a long-term follow-up of 38 patients who had undergone radical surgery for histologically confirmed ASC, the 1-, 2- and 5-year overall survival rates were 34, 11, and 5%, respectively. Furthermore, the authors found that adjuvant chemoradiation (5-FU or gemcitabine or capecitabine plus 5.040 Gy), but not other well-established prognostic determinants (T stage, nodal involvement, residual microscopic tumor), significantly correlated with a better median survival when compared to surgery alone (13.6 vs. 8.6 months respectively; $p = 0.05$). This favorable course was also confirmed in a series from our institution, in which four patients who had undergone pancreatic resection with negative resection margins (R0) plus adjuvant chemotherapy (5-FU, or gemcitabine plus or minus oxaliplatin) had a median survival of 14.5 months (R0; n = 2; 27 months; R1; n = 2; 13.5 months) [4].

Furthermore, alternative treatments such as intraoperative radiation therapy (IORT) for locally advanced ASC and surgery plus adjuvant locoregional chemotherapy also have been reported, although the results are controversial due to the small sample sizes [14, 18, 19]. Therefore, in the absence of further evidence, radical resection of the primary tumor plus adjuvant chemoradiation should be considered the gold standard approach in the multidisciplinary management of ASC.

13.1.4 Prognosis

ASC still represents a particularly aggressive disease associated with poor prognosis. For those patients suffering from locally advanced or metastatic ASC, the median overall survival rate is exceptionally dismal (4.5 months) [8, 11, 14, 20, 21].

Early studies published in the literature failed to document any significant improvement in survival comparing adjuvant chemotherapy with standard resection alone [3, 14, 21, 22]. However, these conclusions might have been biased by the small and heterogeneous samples and the lack of details regarding well-established prognostic factors, such as margin status and TNM stage [3, 8, 21]. Notably, more recent studies, in which detailed surgical and pathological data were included, reported a significantly more favorable outcome within the subset of patients undergoing radical surgery plus adjuvant chemoradiation, with a median overall survival comparable to that of patients with PCs of similar characteristics [5, 11].

13.2 Colloid Carcinoma

Colloid carcinoma is a distinct variant of pancreatic ductal adenocarcinoma, with unique clinical, radiological (Fig. 13.3), and biological characteristics.

Also referred to as mucinous non-cystic carcinoma, colloid carcinoma is almost always observed in association with intestinal-type intraductal papillary mucinous neoplasm (IPMN) and presents macroscopically as a large, well-demarcated gelatinous lesion [23, 24] (Fig. 13.4a). Microscopically, colloid carcinoma is characterized by a paucity of stromal and vascular components and by large pools of mucins, surrounded at least partially by well-dif-

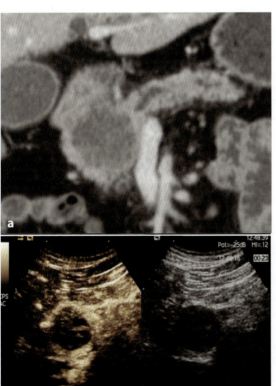

Fig. 13.3 Colloid carcinoma. A hypodense mass in the pancreatic head as seen on CT (**a**) with innervated viable tissue better seen at CEUS (**b**), resulting inhomogeneous vascularization

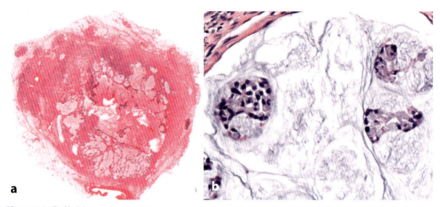

Fig. 13.4 Colloid carcinoma (mucinous non-cystic carcinoma). **a** Gelatinous mass better demarcated than ductal adenocarcinoma. **b** Cluster of cells floating in abundant extracellular mucin

ferentiated cuboidal to columnar neoplastic cells. In addition, clusters of suspended neoplastic cells are observed [23, 24] (Fig. 13.4b).

Colloid carcinomas display intestinal differentiation markers at immunohistochemistry, such as the expression of CK20, MUC2, and CDX2. From a molecular standpoint, these tumors frequently exhibit *KRAS2* and *TP53* mutations, although less frequently than in conventional pancreatic ductal adenocarcinoma [25]. Interestingly, a loss of DCP4/SMAD4 is uncommonly observed in colloid carcinomas. Such biological differences may be responsible for the significantly different behaviors of these tumor types. In fact, recent studies reported the more favorable clinical course and improved long-term survival of patients with colloid carcinoma compared with those with ductal adenocarcinoma [26]. Therefore, a precise recognition at pathologic examination is of paramount importance.

13.3 Medullary Carcinoma of the Pancreas

Medullary carcinomas of the pancreas are a recently described, histologically distinct subset of poorly differentiated adenocarcinomas with a unique pathogenesis and clinical course. This entity, first described in 1998, displays histological characteristics similar to medullary carcinomas observed in other organs, such as the breast and large intestine, i.e., a typical syncytial growth pattern, with poorly differentiated cells, expanding tumor borders without a significant desmoplastic reaction, and T-cell infiltration [27].

From a genetic standpoint, medullary carcinomas are distinct from conventional PC. The majority of these tumors (69%) harbor wild-type K-*RAS* genes, as opposed to pancreatic ductal adenocarcinomas [28]. Also, it has been estimated that one-fourth of all medullary carcinomas display microsatellite instability (MSI) [27], a typical genetic feature but one that is only rarely observed in conventional PC. Thus, standard ductal adenocarcinomas of the pancreas are characterized by genomic instability and chromosomal aberrations [28]. Of note, in the few cases in which MSI was reported, concomitant tumors affecting other organs (more frequently colorectal cancer) but with the same genetic landscape were present, suggesting an inherited basis for the development of these carcinomas.

Remarkably, because of the special genetic, immunohistochemical, and clinical features of medullary carcinoma, recognition of the medullary variant of pancreatic adenocarcinoma is important. Furthermore, an awareness of the distinct histological characteristics of the various forms of PC may be useful to identify an inherited susceptibility to cancer. In such case, any cancer in a first-degree relative of the patient should be carefully investigated.

13.4 Anaplastic Carcinoma

Anaplastic carcinoma is a rare variant, accounting for 5–7% of all pancreatic tumors. It is preferentially located in the tail of the pancreas and it macroscopically appears as a voluminous mass with a variegated aspect on cut section, due to degenerative changes such as necrosis and hemorrhage [29, 30] (Fig. 13.5).

At imaging, anaplastic carcinoma appears as a markedly enhanced mass, with the exception of necrotic areas. Microscopically, it is composed of pleomorphic large cells, giant cells, or spindle cells (Fig. 13.6). The prognosis of

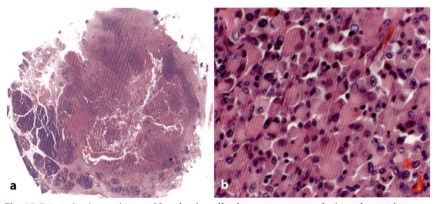

Fig. 13.5 Anaplastic carcinoma. Neoplastic cells show extreme anaplasia and grow in poorly cohesive sheets supported by a scant desmoplastic stroma in this well-demarcated tumor mass with hemorrhagic necrosis

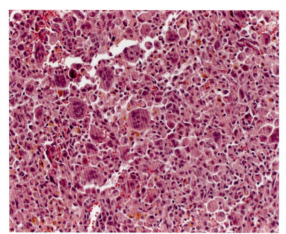

Fig. 13.6 Anaplastic carcinoma, characterized by the presence of non-neoplastic osteoclast-like giant cells

patients with anaplastic carcinoma is worse than that of patients with conventional ductal adenocarcinoma, with distant metastasis frequently present at the time of diagnosis [30].

References

1. Baylor SM, Berg JW (1973) Cross-classification and survival characteristics of 5,000 cases of cancer of the pancreas. J Surg Oncol 5:335-358
2. Cihak RW, Kawashima T, Steer A (1972) Adenoacanthoma (adenosquamous carcinoma) of the pancreas. Cancer 29:1133-1140
3. Madura JA, Jarman BT, Doherty MG et al (1999) Adenosquamous carcinoma of the pancreas. Arch Surg 134:599-603
4. Regi P, Butturini G, Malleo G et al (2011) Clinicopathological features of adenosquamous pancreatic cancer. Langenbecks Arch Surg 396:217-222
5. Voong KR, Davison J, Pawlik TM at al (2010) Resected pancreatic adenosquamous carcinoma: cli nicopathologic review and evaluation of adjuvant chemotherapy and radiation in 38 patients. Hum Pathol 41:113-122
6. Herxheimer G (1907) UberheterologeCancroide. BeitrPatholAnat 41:348-412
7. Klöppel G, Hruban RH, Longnecker DS et al (2000) Tumours of the exocrine pancreas. In: Hamilton SR, Aaltonen LA (eds) World Health Organization classification of tumours. Pathology and genetics of tumours of the digestive system.WHO, Lyon, pp 219-251
8. Kardon DE, Thompson LD, Przygodzki RM, Heffess CS (2001) Adenosquamous carcinoma of the pancreas: a clinicopathologic series of 25 cases. Mod Pathol 14:443-451
9. Chen J, Baithun SI, Ramsay MA (1985) Histogenesis of pancreatic carcinomas: a study based on 248 cases. J Pathol 146:65-76
10. Brody JR, Costantino CL, Potoczek M et al (2009) Adenosquamous carcinoma of the pancreas harbors KRAS2, DPC4 and TP53 molecular alterations similar to pancreatic ductal adenocarcinoma. Mod Pathol 22:651-659
11. Smoot RL, Zhang L, Sebo TJ, Que FG (2008) Adenosquamous carcinoma of the pancreas: a single-institution experience comparing resection and palliative care. J Am Coll Surg 207:368-370

13 Rare Variants of Ductal Adenocarcinoma of the Pancreas

12. Beyer KL, Marshall JB, Metzler MH et al (1992) Squamous cell carcinoma of the pancreas. Report of an unusual case and review of the literature. Dig Dis Sci 37:312-318
13. Itani KM, Karni A, Green L (1999) Squamous cell carcinoma of the pancreas. J Gastrointest Surg 3:512-515
14. Hsu JT, Chen HM, Wu RC et al (2008) Clinicopathologic features and outcomes following surgery for pancreatic adenosquamous carcinoma. World J Surg Oncol 6:95
15. Kobayashi N, Higurashi T, Iida H et al (2008) Adenosquamous carcinoma of the pancreas associated with humoral hypercalcemia of malignancy (HHM). J Hepatobiliary Pancreat Surg 15:531-535
16. Layfield LJ, Cramer H, Madden J et al (2001) Atypical squamous epithelium in cytologic specimens from the pancreas: cytological differential diagnosis and clinical implications. Diagn Cytopathol 25:38-42
17. Lozano MD, Panizo A, Sola IJ, Pardo-Mindan FJ (1998) FNAC guided by computed tomography in the diagnosis of primary pancreatic adenosquamous carcinoma. A report of three cases. Acta Cytol 42:1451-1454
18. Yamaue H, Tanimura H, Onishi H et al (2001) Adenosquamous carcinoma of the pancreas: successful treatment with extended radical surgery, intraoperative radiation therapy, and locoregional chemotherapy. Int J Pancreatol 29:53-58
19. Nabae T, Yamaguchi K, Takahata S et al (1998) Adenosquamous carcinoma of the pancreas: report of two cases. Am J Gastroenterol 93:1167-1170
20. Komatsuda T, Ishida H, Konno K et al (2000) Adenosquamous carcinoma of the pancreas: report of two cases. Abdom Imaging 25:420-423
21. Rahemtullah A, Misdraji J, Pitman MB (2003) Adenosquamous carcinoma of the pancreas: cytologic features in 14 cases. Cancer 99:372-378
22. Yamaguchi K, Enjoji M (1991) Adenosquamous carcinoma of the pancreas: a clinicopathologic study. J Surg Oncol 47:109-116
23. Adsay NV, Pierson C, Sarkar F et al (2001) Colloid (mucinous noncystic) carcinoma of the pancreas. Am J Surg Pathol 25:26-42
24. Seidel G, Zahurak M, Iacobuzio-Donahue C et al (2002) Almost all infiltrating colloid carcinomas of the pancreas and periampullary region arise from in situ papillary neoplasms: a study of 39 cases. Am J Surg Pathol 26:56-63
25. Adsay NV, Merati K, Nassar H et al (2003) Pathogenesis of colloid (pure mucinous) carcinoma of exocrine organs: Coupling of gel-forming mucin (MUC2) production with altered cell polarity and abnormal cell-stroma interaction may be the key factor in the morphogenesis and indolent behavior of colloid carcinoma in the breast and pancreas. Am J Surg Pathol 27:571-578
26. Yopp AC, Katabi N, Janakos M et al (2011) Invasive carcinoma arising in intraductal papillary mucinous neoplasms of the pancreas: a matched control study with conventional pancreatic ductal adenocarcinoma. Ann Surg 253:968-974
27. Wilentz RE, Goggins M, Redston M et al (2000) Genetic, immunohistochemical, and clinical features of medullary carcinoma of the pancreas: A newly described and characterized entity. Am J Pathol 156:1641-1651
28. Goggins M, Offerhaus GJ, Hilgers W et al (1998) Pancreatic adenocarcinomas with DNA replication errors (RER+) are associated with wild-type K-ras and characteristic histopathology. Poor differentiation, a syncytial growth pattern, and pushing borders suggest RER+. Am J Pathol 152:1501-1507
29. Paal E, Thompson LD, Frommelt RA et al (2001) A clinicopathologic and immunohistochemical study of 35 anaplastic carcinomas of the pancreas with a review of the literature. Ann Diagn Pathol 5:129-140
30. Strobel O, Hartwig W, Bergmann F et al (2011) Anaplastic pancreatic carcinoma: Presentation, surgical management, and outcome. Surgery 149:200-208

Rare Primary Tumors of the Pancreas

14

Marco Dal Molin, Paola Capelli, Mirko D'Onofrio,
Ivana Cataldo, Giovanni Marchegiani and Giovanni Butturini

14.1 Acinar Cell Carcinoma

Although pancreatic acinar cells represent > 80% of pancreatic tissue, acinar cell carcinomas (ACCs) account only for 1% of primary pancreatic neoplasms [1-5]. The average age at diagnosis is approximately 60 years old, with the majority of patients being men.

ACC usually presents with non-specific signs or symptoms, such as abdominal pain, weight loss, or an abdominal mass. Occasionally, "Schmid's triad" of subcutaneous fat necrosis, polyarthralgia, and eosinophilia due to increased serum lipase is associated with ACC [5]. In many ACC patients, metastatic disease to the liver and lymph nodes is already present at the time of diagnosis.

ACCs can arise in any portion of the pancreatic gland, although the pancreatic head is more frequently involved. In such cases, as opposed to ductal adenocarcinoma, jaundice is very rare. The tumors are usually large (10 cm on average), well-circumscribed, solid, soft, lesions that on their cut surfaces demonstrate bands of connective tissue circumscribing a nodule of tumor cells, which can have necrotic foci [6] (Fig. 14.1). Some intraductal and cystic subtypes, considered as variants, have also been described.

Microscopically, ACC is a highly cellular neoplasm that lacks the desmoplastic stroma typically observed in pancreatic adenocarcinoma. The characteristic acinar cells (round nuclei and abundant eosinophilic granular PAS-positive cytoplasm) of ACCs grow in solid, trabecular, or glandular patterns, but at least focally the neoplasm shows an acinar architecture with a structurally almost normal appearance (Fig. 14.2).

M. Dal Molin (✉)
Department of Surgery and Oncology, General Surgery Unit, Pancreas Center,
"G.B. Rossi" University Hospital,
Verona, Italy
e-mail: marcodalmo82@gmail.com

P. Pederzoli and C. Bassi (eds.), *Uncommon Pancreatic Neoplasms*,
Updates in Surgery
DOI: 10.1007/978-88-470-2673-5_14, © Springer-Verlag Italia 2013

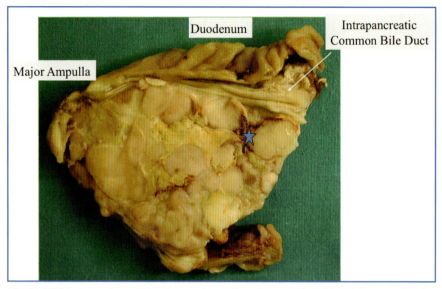

Fig. 14.1 Whipple specimen. Voluminous acinar cell carcinoma with multi-nodular aspect involving extensively the head of the pancreas and dislocating the common bile duct. Foci of necrosis are present (*asterisk*)

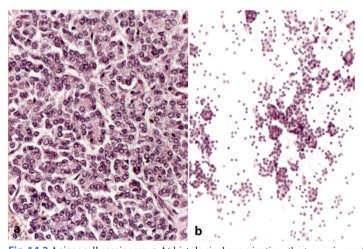

Fig. 14.2 Acinar cell carcinoma. **a** At histological examination, the tumor is mostly characterized by polarized cells resembling acinar cells. An acinar pattern is at least focally present. **b** These features are retained at cytological examination

Immunohistochemistry can be useful in differentiating ACCs from other rare, non-ductal pancreatic tumors, such as neuroendocrine tumors (NETs) [7, 8], by confirming acinar differentiation and variable positivity for pancreatic

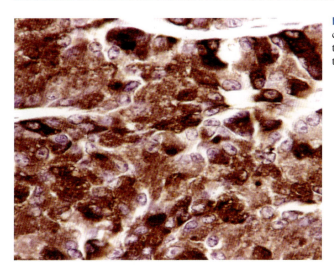

Fig. 14.3 Acinar cell carcinoma: immunohistochemical staining for trypsin

enzymes, especially trypsin, chymotrypsin, and amylase (Fig. 14.3). Recently a new antibody, anti-BCL10, was described as a sensitive and specific marker for acinar cells [9].

At the molecular level, ACCs contain a high frequency of APC/β-catenin pathway mutations; a similar pattern is observed in pancreatoblastomas, as opposed to ductal adenocarcinomas. The most common genetic alteration identified in both ACC and pancreatoblastoma is a loss of heterozygosity involving the short arm of chromosome 11p [10]. Alterations in the β-catenin/APC pathway have also been reported in 50–80% of tumors of this type. Of note, aberrations in the APC/β-catenin pathway result in the nuclear migration of β-catenin, which can be documented at immunohistochemistry [10].

ACC may be associated with elevated serum levels of CEA and CA 19.9, and occasionally with elevated serum AFP (4.5–6% of cases) [11-15].

Pre-operative imaging of ACC is generally non-specific, although a few radiologic patterns have been described. The differential diagnosis of ACC includes ductal adenocarcinoma, NETs, solid pseudopapillary tumors, pancreatoblastoma, mucinous cystic neoplasms, and pseudocysts [16]. Computed tomography (CT) and magnetic resonance imaging (MRI) show cystic areas in 55% of the cases [17]. Chiou et al. described the CT appearance of ACCs as hypodense masses with a well-defined enhancing capsule [18]. Occasionally, intratumoral calcification and necrosis have been reported. Doppler ultrasound (US) examination may facilitate the preoperative differential diagnosis with ductal adenocarcinoma and NENs. The former are usually smaller and clearly hypovascular, while non-functioning NENs are larger and clearly hypervascular at imaging, showing large intralesional vessels on Doppler US [19].

The prognosis of patients with ACCs is generally poor, with median overall survival ranging from 5 to 38 months at different institutions [7, 14, 15, 20-22]. Based upon preoperative imaging, the criteria for tumor resectability are the same as those generally used for ductal adenocarcinoma. Thus, up-front surgery is indicated for resectable ACC. In case of locally advanced ACC or metastatic disease, a neoadjuvant approach has yielded good results. Chemoradiation is generally considered in case of borderline resectable and locally advanced ACC [14, 15]. Therefore, based upon our experience as well a literature review, an aggressive approach is warranted for patients presenting with resectable or locally advanced ACC [23-25]. Reiterative surgery, neoadjuvant and adjuvant chemoradiation therapy, and loco-regional treatment may allow long-term survival and clinical benefit [26-28].

14.2 Pancreatoblastoma

Pancreatoblastoma, originally termed "infantile pancreatic carcinoma" [30], is an extremely rare pancreatic tumor mostly occurring during childhood, although several cases in adults have been described.

In the following, both pediatric and adult pancreatoblastomas are discussed, focusing on their clinical presentation, diagnostic tests, pathologic features, and management.

14.2.1 Pediatric Pancreatoblastoma

Pancreatoblastoma is the most common pancreatic neoplasm of childhood, usually occurring at a median age of 4 years [29-31]. There is a slight male predominance (M:F 1.4:1). Some pancreatoblastomas are seen in association with Beckwith–Weidemann syndrome; all those cases were congenital and characterized by cystic lesions [32]. Typically, patients with pancreatoblastomas present with elevated serum AFP [33].

The clinical presentation of pancreatoblastoma may be heterogeneous. Children with this tumor usually present with upper abdominal pain and often have a palpable epigastric mass [1]. Mechanical obstruction of the duodenum and gastric outlet by the tumor in the head of the pancreas has also been observed. Poor nutritional intake and resultant weight loss are characteristic. Pancreatoblastomas average 10.6 cm in size and develop in the head and tail of the gland with equal frequencies; they are usually well-circumscribed and lobulated [34] (Fig. 14.4).

At histological examination, the tumor consists of large lobules of highly cellular tissue separated by broad fibrous bands. Epithelial cells are arranged in solid sheets, mixed with acinar and occasional semi-glandular structures [34] (Fig. 14.5a). Frequently, the cells tend to form clusters, designated as "squamoid nests" (or squamoid corpuscles), which are a constant and

14 Rare Primary Tumors of the Pancreas

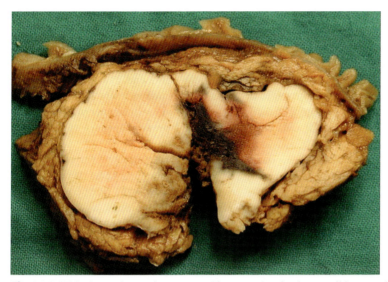

Fig. 14.4. Whipple specimen of a pancreatoblastoma. A voluminous solid mass with clear-cut margins and extensively involving the head of the pancreas. A central hemorrhagic spot is present

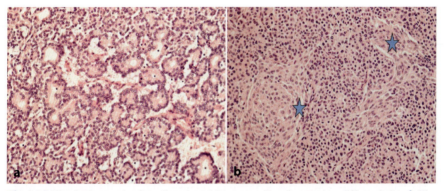

Fig. 14.5 Histologic examination of pancreatoblastoma. **a** Prominent acinar differentiation. **b** The characteristic squamoid corpuscles (*asterisks*)

characteristic features of pancreatoblastomas (Fig. 14.5b). Finally, the stromal bands between the epithelial islands are composed of hypercellular spindle cells with variable collagenization. The stroma is particularly cellular in pediatric pancreatoblastomas, and in rare cases a neoplastic mesenchymal component is present [34, 35].

Most often, the molecular alterations involve the β-catenin gene, as discussed previously.

Imaging techniques, such as CT, performed for abdominal pain or other symptoms, or less frequently for unrelated reasons, can show a large, finely calcified mass in the pancreas. Usually, both solid and cystic elements are present, and foci of hemorrhagic necrosis are not infrequently seen [36, 37].

The differential diagnosis includes other solid, cellular neoplasms of the pancreas, such as acinar cell carcinomas, solid pseudopapillary tumors, and NETs [38, 39].

One-third of patients with pancreatoblastomas already present with metastases at the time of diagnosis, while in other patients metastases develop later, as a consequence of tumor progression [34]. The liver is the most common site of metastases, followed by the regional lymph nodes, lungs, and peritoneum [34, 40].

The best treatment for localized tumors in pediatric patients is complete surgical resection, which in these cases is usually curative. Children with metastatic disease generally have a fairly poor prognosis, although in more recent reports favorable responses to chemotherapy and radiation were obtained [41], suggesting that in selected cases long-term survival can be achieved.

14.2.2 Pancreatoblastoma in Adults

In adults, as in children, the differential diagnosis of pancreatoblastoma includes non-functioning pancreatic NETs, acinar cell carcinoma, solid pseudopapillary tumor, and ductal adenocarcinoma. Non-functioning pancreatic NETs typically present with elevated chromogranin A [38, 42]. Solid-pseudopapillary tumors are usually well-demarcated, large, and often heterogeneous masses that may contain peripheral calcifications. However, aggressive behavior is rarely observed in these tumors. Furthermore, solid-pseudopapillary tumors do not have central calcifications, are mainly seen in young females, and are predominantly cystic. In addition, they do not express AFP, the production of which is closely linked to acinar differentiation [38, 42]. These features may be helpful in distinguishing solid-pseudopapillary tumors from pancreatoblastoma.

In adults and in children, surgical resection is the best curative option to for maximum long-term survival [43-48]. However, curative resection is not always feasible, due to metastatic presentation at the time of diagnosis, which occurs in approximately 25% of patients [34, 43-48]. The reported median survival rate in adults is 18.5 months.

The role of adjuvant therapy after surgical treatment is unclear and mostly based on the preference of single institutions. Some authors have strongly advocated the use adjuvant chemotherapy because of the malignant features of pancreatoblastoma [34, 40].

Given its rarity, the natural history of adult pancreatoblastoma and the prognosis of these patients are poorly understood. In our report of adult patients with this tumor [43], the very long disease-free interval after resection (51 months) in one of the two patients in the series, underscores the efficacy of aggressive surgical treatment as a determinant factor in long-term survival. Notably, no adjuvant therapy was necessary in that particular patient.

14.3 Primary Pancreatic Lymphoma

Primary pancreatic lymphoma is rare, comprising < 0.5% of pancreatic tumors [49]. These patients usually present with symptoms of carcinoma of the pancreatic head. An accurate cytopathologic diagnosis by fine-needle aspiration (FNA) (Fig. 14.6) is of paramount importance because the primary treatment is non-surgical, based on a combination of chemotherapy and radiation therapy.

14.3.1 Clinical Presentation

Abdominal lymphoma, which is typically a non-Hodgkin's lymphoma (NHL), involves extranodal tissues in up to 40% of patients. Furthermore, the gastrointestinal tract, particularly the stomach and small bowel, are the most commonly involved extranodal sites [50]. Primary localization of the NHL in the pancreas is rare and accounts for < 0.5% of all pancreatic malignancies and 1% of all extranodal lymphomas [51, 52].

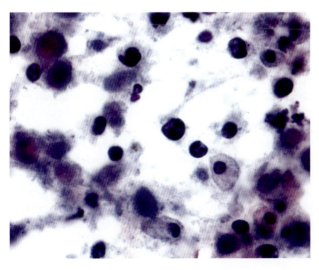

Fig. 14.6 Large-cell lymphoma of the pancreas, showing large atypical interspersed lymphoid cells

Primary pancreatic lymphoma is often described as a large, homogeneous mass in the head of the pancreas, with signs of extension outside the gland, with or without associated lymphadenopathy. Less common pancreatic presentations are body or tail masses or, more rarely, involvement of the entire gland [52].

Pancreatic lymphoma may initially mimic pancreatic adenocarcinoma: symptoms at the time of diagnosis include abdominal pain, jaundice, acute pancreatitis, weight loss, and nausea and vomiting. However, involvement of the lymph nodes or other organs is usually present, questioning the diagnosis of pancreatic cancer [53]. Interestingly, the classical symptoms of lymphoma, such as fever and night sweats, are rarely observed. Abdominal pain, unlike adenocarcinoma, rarely radiates to the back [54, 55].

14.3.2 Diagnosis

Although specific biochemical markers for primary pancreatic lymphoma are not available, elevated serum LDH and α2-microglobulin have been shown to be of important diagnostic and prognostic value. In the case of a large mass in the head of the pancreas without biliary obstruction, pain, or weight loss, an elevated serum LDH level helps clarify the diagnosis [55]. CA 19.9 is usually normal, unless biliary obstruction is present. Elevated serum soluble interleukin-2 receptor (sIL-2R) levels have been reported in both hematologic and non-hematologic solid neoplasms. While elevated levels of sIL-2R have not been shown to be associated with cancer, values > 5000 U/ml may are suggestive in the presence of rounded pancreatic lesions [56].

Abdominal ultrasound may show a large, bulky, homogeneous, hypoechoic lesion associated with peri-pancreatic and peri-aortic lymphadenopathy, highly suggestive of the hematologic nature of the disease [57].

CT is usually the method of choice to evaluate a pancreatic solid mass. Pancreatic lymphoma can present as a well-defined mass or as a large infiltrating lesion with poorly defined contours. Most pancreatic lymphomas show homogeneous enhancement after intravenous injection of contrast medium, which helps to discriminate them from more commonly observed adenocarcinomas. The combination of the above-cited characteristics, the absence of dilatation of the main pancreatic duct, and concomitant retroperitoneal lymphadenopathy suggest a diagnosis of lymphoma [58-61].

Positron emission tomography is generally useful in the staging of lymphoma, particularly in differentiating lymphoma from ductal adenocarcinoma [62].

Preoperative tissue sampling should always be performed if lymphoma is suspected, to confirm the diagnosis. Endoscopic US-guided FNA biopsy with flow cytometric analysis is helpful. Despite these sensitive techniques, preoperative diagnosis is still difficult to achieve in most patients (72%) [63-65].

14.3.3 Treatment

For more than 30 years, the treatment of NHL has been based on chemotherapy and radiotherapy regimens. Surgery has been generally restricted to tissue procurement for diagnosis. Behrns et al. retrospectively evaluated 12 patients with pancreatic lymphoma who underwent radiation therapy and/or chemotherapy in a single institution [52]. Ten of those patients (83.3%), all of whom eventually died of progressive lymphoma, received radiation therapy and/or chemotherapy, and no patient remained disease-free at follow-up. Mean survival was 13 months for patients who received chemotherapy alone (n = 2), 22 months for those treated with radiation therapy only (n = 5), and 26 months for those receiving combined radiation therapy and chemotherapy (n = 3).

The most common chemotherapy regimens include CVP (cis-platinum, vincristine, and peplomycin) and CHOP (cyclophosphamide, hydroxyl-daunorubicin (doxorubicin), oncovin (vincristine), prednisone). The addition of rituximab to the CHOP regimen was shown to increase the complete response rate and to prolong overall survival in patients with diffuse large-B-cell lymphoma, without a significant increase in toxicity [66]

The role of radiation therapy in management is not well defined, although local radiotherapy up to a total of 40 Gy has been used as consolidation after chemotherapy [67].

14.4 Hepatoid Carcinoma

Pancreatic hepatoid carcinomas are extrahepatic neoplasms exhibiting morphologic and immunohistochemical features of hepatocellular carcinomas [68] (Fig. 14.7). They represent an extremely uncommon group of tumors: to date, fewer than 20 have been reported [69, 70]. They can present in pure forms or in association with other morphological aspects, such as NETs or ductal adenocarcinomas [71]. The biological behavior of the pure forms seems to be more indolent than that of heterogeneous tumors.

The hepatoid component accounts for the histological features of an expansive tumor composed of large eosinophilic or clear cells, sometimes with granular cytoplasm, growing in a sheet-like or trabecular pattern with sinusoidal vascular channels. Abundant cytoplasmic glycogen, hyaline globules, and especially bile production are other diagnostic features (Fig. 14.8). Although not specific, hepatoid carcinomas are also characterized by AFP production which, apart from a few negative examples, can be detected in the serum or in tumor cells by immunohistochemistry in most cases [72].

Even when preoperative correct diagnosis cannot be reached mainly due to rarity and non-specific imaging features, surgical excision based on typical pancreatic resections may yield good long-term results, but further studies and longer follow up are needed to correctly assess the prognostic features of these tumors.

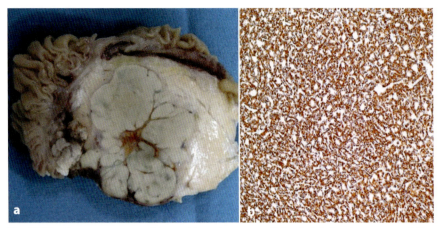

Fig. 14.7 a Gross appearance of hepatoid carcinoma; a solid poly-lobulated mass, resembling hepatocellular carcinoma. **b** Immunohistochemical staining for hepatocyte paraffin-1 antibody

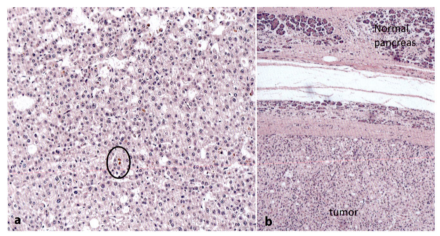

Fig. 14.8 Pancreatic hepatoid tumor. **a** Neoplasm with solid-nested-trabecular architecture; in this case, bile pigment is present (*circled*). **b** The tumor is well demarcated from the normal pancreas

14.5 Granular Cell Tumor

Granular-cell tumor (GCT) is a rare histotype, first described in 1926 by Abrikossoff. These tumors arise in a large variety of organs (tongue, oral mucosa, skin, and subcutaneous tissue, breast, thyroid, respiratory tract, biliary tree, female genital tract, nervous system, and all segments of the gastrointestinal tract). Only five cases of GCT of the pancreas have been reported to date [73, 74].

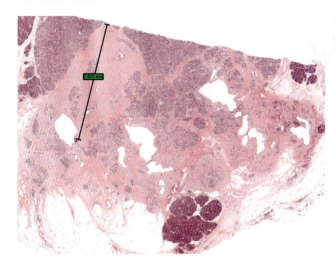

Fig. 14.9 Pancreatic granular-cell tumor; solid lesion approaching the duct of Wirsung

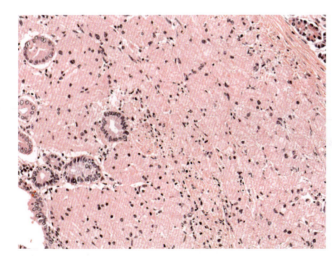

Fig. 14.10 Granular-cell tumor at histological examination. The tumor is characterized by cells with abundant eosinophilic granular cytoplasm; the pattern is pseudoinfiltrative, with clusters of acinar cells and small pancreatic ducts admixed with the tumor cells

The diagnostic work-up may be misleading. In our patient, a cystic lesion in the tail of the pancreas pancreas was determined, initially interpreted as a mucinous tumor. After surgical resection, a white nodular area approximately 8 mm in diameter was macroscopically present in the specimen. This lesion had caused narrowing of the main pancreatic duct and cystic dilation of a branch duct (Fig. 14.9).

Microscopically, a light, partially fringed nodule made up of large clusters of eosinophilic cells with small nuclei and abundant cytoplasm is seen (Figs. 14.10,

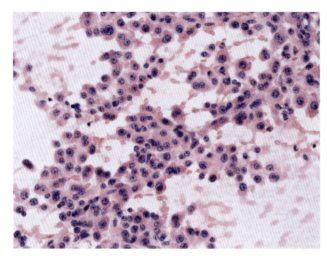

Fig. 14.11 Granular-cell carcinoma at cytologic examination. Polygonal-shaped cells with granular eosinophilic cytoplasm and nuclei with prominent nucleoli are seen on this smear

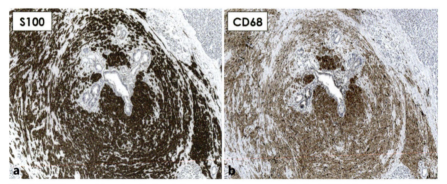

Fig. 14.12 Immunohistochemical staining of granular tumor cells for S100 (**a**) e CD68 (**b**)

14.11). Neoplastic cells stain positively for CK8/18, NSE, S100, and CD68, thereby confirming the diagnosis of GCT [73, 75] (Fig. 14.12).

14.6 Germ-cell Tumors of the Pancreas

Germ-cell tumors occasionally involve the pancreas. Mature teratoma (also known as dermoid cyst of the pancreas) is an extremely rare, benign germ-cell neoplasm, with only a handful of primary pancreatic cases reported in the literature [76]. The differential diagnosis of these lesions includes other pancreatic cystic neoplasms, and the final verdict is usually dictated by pathologic examination.

14.7 Sugar Tumors

Sugar tumors belong to the perivascular epithelioid-cell neoplasms (PEComas) family. To date, only a few PEComas have been reported in the pancreas. These are well-vascularized neoplasms composed of large, clear, epithelioid smooth muscle cells. They variably express HMB45 and smooth-muscle actin but not keratins [77, 78].

References

1. Chen J, Baithum SI (1985) Morphological study of 391 cases of exocrine pancreatic tumours with special reference to the classification of exocrine pancreatic carcinoma. J Pathol 146:17-29
2. Cubilla AL, Fitzgerald PJ (1975) Morphological patterns of primary nonendocrine human pancreas. Cancer Res 35:2234-2238
3. Cubilla AL, Fitzgerald PJ (1979) Cancer of the pancreas (nonendocrine): A suggested morphological classification. Semin Oncol 6:285-297
4. Morohoshi T, Held G, Kloppel G (1983) Exocrine pancreatic tumours and their histological classification: A study based on 167 autopsy and 97 surgical cases. Histopathology 7:645-661
5. Ordonez NG (2001) Pancreatic acinar cell carcinoma. Adv Anat Pathol 8:144-159
6. Basturk O, Zamboni G, Klimstra DS et al (2007) Intraductal and papillary variants of acinar cell carcinomas. Am J Surg Pathol 31:363-370
7. Holen KD, Klimstra DS, Hummer A et al (2002) Clinical characteristic and outcomes from an institutional series of acinar cell carcinoma of the pancreas and related tumours. J Clin Oncol 20:4673-4678
8. Seth AK, Argani P, Campbell KA et al (2008) Acinar cell carcinoma of the pancreas: an institutional series of resected patients and review of the current literature. J Gastrointestinal Surg 12:1061-1067
9. La Rosa S, Franzi F, Marchet S et al (2009) The monoclonal anti-BCL10 antibody (clone 331.1) is a sensitive and specific marker of pancreatic acinar cell carcinoma and pancreatic metaplasia. Virchows Arch 454:133-142
10. Lowery MA, Klimstra DS, Shia J et al (2011) Acinar cell carcinoma of the pancreas: new genetic and treatment insights into a rare malignancy. Oncologist 16:1714-1720
11. Kitagami H, Kondo S, Hirano S et al (2007) Acinar cell carcinoma of the Pancreas. Clinical analysis of 115 patients from pancreatic cancer registry of Japan Pancreas Society. Pancreas 35:42-46
12. Klimstra DS, Heffess CS, Oertel JE, Rosai J (1992) Acinar cell carcinoma of the pancreas. A clinicopahologic study of 28 cases. Am J Surg Pathol 16:815-837
13. Cingolani N, Shaco-Levy R, Farruggio A et al (2000) Alpha-fetoprotein production by pancreatic tumours exhibiting acinar cell differentiation: study of five cases, one arising in a mediastinal teratoma. Hum Pathol 31:938-944
14. Eriguchi N, Aoyagi S, Hara M et al (2000) Large acinar cell carcinoma of the pancreas in a patient with elevated serum AFP level. L Hepatobiliary Pancreatic Surg 7:222-225
15. Chen CP, Chao Y, Li CP et al (2001) Concurrent Chemoradiation is effective in the treatment of alpha-fetoprotein-producing acinar cell carcinoma of the pancreas: report of a case. Pancreas 22:326-329
16. Solcia E, Capella C, Kloppel G (1997) Tumours of the exocrine pancreas. In Rosai J, Sorbin L (eds) Atlas of tumour pathology. 3rd series, fasc. 20. Armed Forces Institute of Pathology, Washington, DC, pp 31-144
17. Tatli S, Mortele KJ, Levy AD et al (2005) CT and MRI features of pure acinar cell carcinoma. Am J Roentgenol 184:511-519

18. Chiou YY, Chiang Jh, Hwang JI et al (2004) Acinar cell carcinoma of the pancreas: clinical and computer tomography manifestation. J Comput Assist Tomogr 28:180-186
19. D'Onofrio M, Mansueto G, Falconi M et al (2004) Neuroendocrine pancreatic tumour: value of contrast enhanced ultrasonography. Abdom Imaging 29:246-258
20. Schmidt CM, Matos JM, Bentrem DJ et al (2008) Acinar cell carcinoma of the pancreas in the United States: prognostic factors and comparison to ductal adenocarcinoma. J Gastrointest Surg 12:2078-2086
21. Matos JM, Schmidt CM, Turrini O et al (2009) Pancreatic Acinar cell carcinoma: a multi-institutional study. J Gastrointest Surg 13:1495-502
22. Wisnoski NC, Townsend CM Jr., Nealon WH et al (2008) 672 patients with acinar cell carcinoma of the pancreas: a population-based comparison to pancreatic adenocarcinoma. Surgery 144:141-148
23. Lee JL, Kim TW, Chang HM et al (2003) Locally advanced acinar cell carcinoma of the pancreas successfully trrated by capecitabine and concurrent radiotherapy: report of two cases. Pancreas 27:e18-e22
24. Kobayashi S, Ishikawa O, Ohigashi H et al (2001) Acinar cell carcinoma of the pancreas treated by en bloc resection and intraperitoneal chemotherapy for peritoneal relapse: a case report of a 15-year survivor. Pancreas 23:109-112
25. Antoine M, Khitrik-Palchuk M, Saif MW (2007) Long-term survival in a patient with acinar cell carcinoma of the Pancreas. A case report and review of literature. J Pancreas 8:783-89
26. Klimstra DS (2007) Nonductal neoplasms of the pancreas. Mod Pathol 20:94-112
27. Lowery MA, Klimstra DS, Shia J et al (2011) Acinar cell carcinoma of the pancreas: new genetic and treatment insights into a rare malignancy. Oncologist 16:1714-1720
28. Yamamoto T, Ohzato H, Fukunaga M et al (2012) Acinar cell carcinoma of the pancreas: a possible role of S-1 as chemotherapy for acinar cell carcinoma. A case report. J Pancreas 13:87-90
29. Becker WF (1957) Pancreatoduodenectomy for carcinoma of the pancreas in an infant; report of a case. Ann Surg 145:864-870
30. Kissane JM (1994) Pancreatoblastoma and solid and cystic papillary tumor: two tumors related to pancreatic ontogeny. Semin Diagn Pathol 11:152-164
31. Horie A, Yano Y, Kotoo Y, Miwa A (1977) Morphogenesis of pancreatoblastoma, infantile carcinoma of the pancreas: report of two cases. Cancer Jan 39:247-254
32. Kerr NJ, Fukuzawa R, Reeve AE, Sullivan MJ (2002) Beckwith-Wiedemann syndrome, pancreatoblastoma, and the wnt signaling pathway. Am J Pathol 160:1541-1542
33. Dhebri AR, Connor S, Campbell F et al (2004) Diagnosis, treatment and outcome of pancreatoblastoma. Pancreatology 4:441-451
34. Klimstra DS, Wenig BM, Adair CF, Heffess CS (1995) Pancreatoblastoma. A clinicopathologic study and review of the literature. Am J Surg Pathol 19:1371-1389
35. Solcia E, Capella C, Kloppel G. PB (1997) In: Rosai J, Sobin LH (eds) Tumors of the pancreas. Atlas of tumour pathology. Armed Forces Institute of Pathology, Washington, DC, pp. 114–9
36. Mergo PJ, Helmberger TK, Buetow PC et al (1997) Pancreatic neoplasms: MR imaging and pathologic correlation. RadioGraphics 17:281-301
37. Roebuck DJ, Yuen MK, Wong YC et al (2001) Imaging features of pancreatoblastoma. Pediatr Radiol 31:501-506
38. Dong PR, Lu DS, Degregario F et al (1996) Solid and papillary neoplasm of the pancreas: radiological-pathological study of five cases and review of the literature. Clin Radiol 51:702-705
39. Klimstra DS, Heffes CS, Oertl J, Rosai J (1992) Acinar cell carcinoma of the pancreas. A clinicopathologic study of 28 cases. Am J Surg Pathol 16:815-837
40. Saif MW (2007) Pancreatoblastoma. JOP 8:55-63
41. Défachelles AS, Martin De Lassalle E, Boutard P et al (2001) Pancreatoblastoma in childhood: clinical course and therapeutic management of seven patients. Med Pediatr Oncol 37:47-52
42. Ohtomo K, Furui S, Onoue M et al (1992) Solid and papillary epithelial neoplasm of the pancreas: MR imaging and pathologic correlation. Radiology 184:567-570

14 Rare Primary Tumors of the Pancreas

43. Cavallini A, Falconi M, Bortesi L et al (2009) Pancreatoblastoma in adults: a review of the literature. Pancreatology 9:73-80
44. Levey JM, Banner BF (1996) Adult pancreatoblastoma: a case report and review of the literature. Am J Gastroenterol 91:1841-1844
45. Montemarano H, Lonergan GJ, Bulas DI, Selby DM (2000) Pancreatoblastoma: imaging findings in 10 patients and review of the literature. Radiology 214:476-482
46. Rajpal S, Warren RS, Alexander M et al (2006) Pancreatoblastoma in an adult: case report and review of the literature. J Gastrointest Surg 10:829-836
47. Dunn JL, Longnecker DS (1995) Pancreatoblastoma in an older adult. Arch Pathol Lab Med 119:547-551
48. Palosaari D, Clayton F, Seaman J (1986) Pancreatoblastoma in an adult. Arch Pathol Lab Med 110:650-652
49. Baylor SM, Berg JW (1973) Cross-classification and survival characteristics of 5,000 cases of cancer of the pancreas. J Surg Oncol 5:335-358
50. Zucca E, Roggero E, Bertoni F et al (1997) Primary extranodal non-Hodgkin's lymphomas. Part 1: gastrointestinal, cutaneous and genitourinary lymphomas. Ann Oncol 8:727-737
51. Freeman C, Berg JW, Cutler SJ (1972) Occurence and prognosis of extra nodal lymphomas. Cancer 29:252-260
52. Salvatore JR, Cooper B, Shah I (2000) Primary pancreatic lymphomas: a case report, literature review and proposal for nomenclature. Med Oncol 17:237-247
53. Federico E, Falconi M, Zuodar G (2011) B-cell lymphoma presenting as acute pancreatitis. Pancreatology 11:553-556
54. Fernandez-del Castillo C, Jimenez RE (2002) Pancreatic cancer, cystic pancreatic neoplasms, and other nonendocrine pancreatic tumours. In: Feldman M, Friedman LS, Sleisenger MH, eds. Sleisenger & Fordtran's gastrointestinal and liver disease, 7th edn. Saunders, Philadelphia, PA, pp. 970-987
55. Cooper D (2004) Tumour markers. In: Goldman L, Ausiello D (eds) Cecil textbook of medicine, 22nd edn. Saunders, Philadelphia, PA, pp. 1131-1134
56. Matsubayashi H, Takagaki S, Otsubo T et al (2002) Pancreatic T-cell lymphoma with high level of soluble interleukin-2 receptor. J Gastroenterol 37:863-867
57. Cario E, Runzi M, Metz K et al (1997) Diagnostic dilemma in pancreatic lymphoma. Int J Pancreatol 22:67-71
58. Prayer L, Schurawitzki H, Mallek R (1992) CT in pancreatic involvement of non-Hodgkin lymphoma. Acta Radiol 33:123-127
59. Van Beers B, Lalonde L, Soyer P et al (1997) Dynamic CT in pancreatic lymphoma. J Comput Assist Tomogr 17:94-97
60. Teefey SA, Stephens DH, Sheedy PF (1986) 2nd CT appearance of primary pancreatic lymphoma. Gastrointest Radiol 11:41-43
61. Merkle EM, Bender GN, Brambs HJ (2000) Imaging findings in pancreatic lymphoma. AJR Am J Roentgenol 174:671-675
62. Yoon SN, Lee MH, Yoon JK (2004) F-18 FDG positron emission tomography findings in primary pancreatic lymphoma. Clin Nucl Med 29:574-575
63. Brown PC, Hart MJ, White TT (1987) Pancreatic lymphoma, diagnosis and management. Int J Pancreatol 2:93-99
64. Nayer H, Weir EG, Sheth S (2004) Primary pancreatic lymphomas: a cytopathologic analysis of a rare malignancy. Cancer 102:315-321
65. Behrns KE, Sarr MG, Strickler JG (1994) Pancreatic lymphoma: is it a surgical disease? Pancreas 9:662-667
66. Pfreundschuh M, Trümper L, Osterborg A et al; MabThera International Trial Group (2006) CHOP-like chemotherapy plus rituximab versus CHOP-like chemotherapy alone in young patients with good-prognosis diffuse large-B-cell lymphoma: a randomised controlled trial by the MabThera International Trial (MInT) Group. Lancet Oncol 7:379-391.
67. Shahar KH, Carpenter LS, Jorgensen J (2005) Role of radiation therapy in a patient with primary pancreatic lymphoma. Clin Lymphoma Myeloma 6:143-145

68. Ishikura H, Fukasawa Y, Ogasawara K et al (1985) An AFP-producing gastric carcinoma with features of hepatic differentiation. A case report. Cancer 56:840-848
69. Hameed O, Haodong X, Saddeghi S et al (2007) Hepatoid carcinoma of the pancreas: a case report and literature review of a heterogeneous group of tumors. Am J Surg Pathol 31:146-152
70. Hughes K, Kelty S, Martin R (2004) Hepatoid carcinoma of the pancreas. Am Surg 70:1030-1033
71. Jung JY, Kim YJ, Kim HM et al (2010) Hepatoid carcinoma of the pancreas combined with neuroendocrine carcinoma. Gut Liver 4:98-102
72. Brandi G, Nobili E, Capizzi E et al (2008) Exocrine-endocrine pancreatic cancer and alpha-fetoprotein. Pancreas 37:223-225
73. Kanno A, Satoh K, Hirota M et al (2010) Granular cell tumor of the pancreas: A case report and review of literature. World J Gastrointest Oncol 2:121-124
74. Seidler A, Burstein S, Drweiga W, Goldberg M (1986) Granular cell tumor of the pancreas. J Clin Gastroenterol 8:207-209
75. Cavaliere A, Sidoni A, Ferri I, Falini B (1994) Granular cell tumor: an immunohistochemical study. Tumori 80:224-228
76. Singhi AD, Hruban RH, Fabre M et al (2011) Peripancreatic paraganglioma: a potential diagnostic challenge in cytopathology and surgical pathology. Am J Surg Pathol 35:1498-1504
77. Hirabayashi K, Nakamura N, Kajiwara H et al (2009) Perivascular epithelioid cell tumor (PEComa) of the pancreas: immunoelectron microscopy and review of the literature. Pathol Int 59:650-655
78. Zamboni G, Pea M, Martignoni G et al (1996) Clear cell "sugar" tumor of the pancreas. A novel member of the family of lesions characterized by the presence of perivascular epithelioid cells. Am J Surg Pathol 20:722-730

Rare Secondary Tumors of the Pancreas 15

Giovanni Butturini, Marco Inama, Marco Dal Molin,
Mirko D'Onofrio, Davide Melisi, Giampaolo Tortora,
Federica Pedica and Paola Capelli

15.1 Introduction

Secondary neoplasms involving the pancreas are less common than primary neoplasms. The pancreas is rarely the only metastatic site and metastases can reach the pancreas by lymphatic or hematogenous routes. Several tumors have been demonstrated to metastasize to the pancreas; however, there are differences in the prevalence of the various tumor types that colonize the pancreas, depending upon the population considered (autopsy records vs. surgical specimens).

The most common primary tumors that metastasize to the pancreas are renal cell carcinomas (RCCs), lung cancer, breast cancer, malignant melanoma, carcinomas of the gastrointestinal tract, and prostate cancer. In addition, almost all hematopoietic neoplasms can involve the pancreas and on rare occasions occur as an isolated mass. Among these, non-Hodgkin lymphoma is the most common [1].

15.2 Clinicopathological Features of Pancreatic Metastases

Pancreatic metastases rarely occur as an isolated focus, rather as disseminated disease. In fact, autopsy and surgical series report an incidence of pancreatic metastases between 1.6% and 11% [2-4]. When a pancreatic mass is detected, the incidence of a secondary tumor increases to > 40% if the patient had a previously diagnosed non-pancreatic neoplasm [5, 6].

G. Butturini (✉)
Department of Surgery and Oncology, General Surgery Unit, Pancreas Center,
"G.B. Rossi" University Hospital,
Verona, Italy
e-mail: giovanni.butturini@ospedaleuniverona.it

P. Pederzoli and C. Bassi (eds.), *Uncommon Pancreatic Neoplasms*,
Updates in Surgery
DOI: 10.1007/978-88-470-2673-5_15, © Springer-Verlag Italia 2013

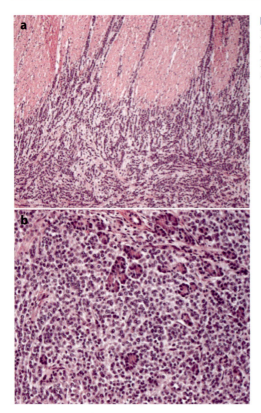

Fig. 15.1 Metastatic breast cancer. Histologically, the neoplastic cells involve the duodenal wall (a) and pancreatic lobules, replacing normal acinar tissue (b)

Due to improvements in the diagnostic process, the recognition of pancreatic metastasis has improved, such that pancreatic metastasectomies have been reported to account for around 4% of all pancreatic resections [7]. The most common metastatic cancer to the pancreas as determined in surgical specimens is clear-cell renal carcinoma, but other tumors seem to have a particular affinity for the gland, such as breast cancer (Fig. 15.1), lung cancer, melanoma, sarcoma, colon cancer, and endometrial carcinoma [5]. Still, the exact prevalence of pancreatic metastatic tumors is unknown and a certain discrepancy exists between surgical and autopsy series. For example, Adsay et al. [2] studied 190 autopsy cases involving pancreatic tumors, 43% of which were secondary tumors. Most of them were of epithelial origin, most commonly from the lung (42%), gastrointestinal tract (24.7%), kidney (5%), breast (3.7%), liver (2.5%), ovary (1.2%), and urinary bladder (1.2%). All tumors in that study presented as disseminated disease.

With regard to the location, 25% of the metastatic tumors were confined to the head of the pancreas, with one case involving the body and six occurring in the tail, but the vast majority of the tumors (75%) involved multiple segments of the organ.

A recent surgical literature review of 220 patients (Table 15.1) demonstrated that most pancreatic metastases are RCCs (70.5%), followed by breast (6.8%), lung

Table 15.1 Pathology, symptoms, and type of surgery for cancer metastatic to the pancreas, as reported in the literature (n = 220 patients)

Pathology	Percentage
Renal cell cancer	70.5
Lung cancer	5.9
Breast cancer	6.8
Colorectal cancer	5.5
Melanoma	2.7
Others	8.6
Symptoms[a]	
None	27.6
Jaundice	25.2
Pain	19.7
Weight loss	10.2
Gastrointestinal bleeding	11
Pancreatitis	4.7
Other	17.3
Surgical procedure	
Pancreaticoduodenectomy	40%
Distal pancreatectomy	20.9
Total pancreatectomy	15
Other	24.1

[a]Some patients had more than one symptom.

(5.9%), and colorectal (5.5%) tumors, and melanoma (2.7%) [3]. Carcinomas of the gastrointestinal tract most often involve the pancreas "ab estrinseco," by direct extension (such as carcinomas of the ampulla of Vater, extrahepatic bile ducts, duodenum, and stomach). Lymphatic dissemination is generally the diffusion modality of colorectal cancer, due to the unique lymphatic drainage through the mesocolon to the pancreas. In such cases, the most frequent site of implantation of metastatic cells is the inferior portion of the head of the pancreas.

Histologically, metastases usually involve the pancreatic lobules expanding the interlobular septa, replacing normal acinar tissue. Clusters of acinar cells and small pancreatic ducts entrapped within the tumor cells are often observed. This pattern of growth, although not exclusive to metastases, is suggestive of a secondary lesion, especially when a primary pancreatic tumor has been excluded. Nevertheless, secondary tumors of the pancreas can represent a diagnostic challenge, not only from a clinical standpoint but also histopathologically. Remarkably, in the above-mentioned autopsy study [2], lymphomas, melanomas, and sarcomas were difficult to distinguish from anaplastic pancreatic carcinomas. Radiologically and at gross examination, metastases can mimic primary tumors of the pancreas, especially when they present as solitary masses. As a result, solitary metastases can be diagnostically challenging, and detailed knowledge of the patient's medical history is crucial. A correct diagnosis is extremely important since patients with metastatic disease to the pancreas generally have different therapeutic options than those with a primary pancreatic tumor. Morphological evidence of a metastatic neoplasm can be obtained with fine-needle aspiration (FNA) cytology. The histological diagnosis relies on the presence of distinctive features, for example melanin pigment in melanomas (Figs. 15.2, 15.3) and a known history of a previously treated non-pancreatic neoplasm (e.g., RCC).

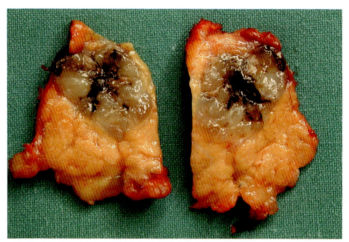

Fig. 15.2 Metastatic melanoma to the pancreas. Solid mass with black to brown area reflecting the presence of melanin pigment

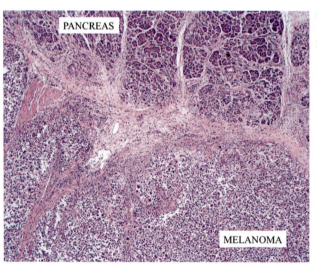

Fig. 15.3 Metastatic melanoma and normal pancreas

15.3 Renal Cell Carcinoma Metastatic to the Pancreas

Among isolated pancreatic metastases those arising from renal cell carcinomas (RCCs), the most common histotype in this patient subgroup [7], are frequently resectable. This is due to the relatively indolent course of metastatic RCC in the pancreas. In the past, some authors recommended the conservative management of these patients, reporting good survival results [8] or in some cases spontaneous regression of the disease [9]. However, RCC pancreatic metastases can be associated with synchronus extrapancreatic disease. In such patients the prognosis is dismal [10].

The mechanism of metastatization is still unclear. The average 10-year delay from primary RCC resection to metachronous isolated pancreatic metastases offers no explanation, as yet. Most specimens of pancreatic RCC metastases are N0 [11], so that it is difficult to argue a lymphogenous origin of the secondary tumor. At the same time, there is no correlation between the site of the primary and that of the pancreatic mass, seemingly ruling out a mechanism invoking local invasion or implantation during primary RCC resection [12, 13]. Current research interest is therefore focused on the high affinity of RCC cells for the pancreatic parenchyma. New insights into cellular cross-talk could clarify the specific behavior of RCC metachronous metastases [14].

15.3.1 Clinical Presentation

Due to their expansive growth pattern, isolated RCC pancreatic metastases produce specific symptoms only when the size of the tumor is quite large. In these patients, the clinical presentation may include gastrointestinal bleeding and anemia due to the hypervascularity of the lesions and, consequently, erosion of the duodenal wall, jaundice, or duodenal obstruction. Rarer symptoms of pancreatic insufficiency, palpable tumor, and pancreatitis have been described. Other, generic symptoms are fatigue, weight loss, and abdominal pain. Serum tumor markers are generally within the limits, as is the case with other metastatic diseases in the pancreas [15-19].

However, almost half of the patients are asymptomatic at diagnosis and the pancreatic lesions are discovered by ultrasound (US) during a routine program of follow-up after RCC resection, or for other non-specific abdominal complaints following surgery for RCC even if it occurred many years earlier [19]. This is consistent with the typically long interval between RCC primary resection and pancreatic metastases, which according to reports is 10 years on average but as long as 32.7 years [13, 17, 20-23]. Consequently a yearly abdominal US examination is strongly recommended for all patients with a history of resected RCC, and a pancreatic metastasis should be considered as the first diagnostic likelihood whenever a hypervascularized tumor in the pancreas is detected.

15.3.2 Diagnostic Work-up

Typically, hypervascular, pancreatic metastases from RCC can be characterized by dynamic imaging, which easily rules out a differential diagnosis of pancreatic ductal adenocarcinoma [24, 25]. However, the imaging features of pancreatic metastases from RCC cannot be differentiated from those of neuroendocrine tumors (NETs). The differential diagnosis is therefore based on the clinical history and symptoms, including a correlation with a specific hypersecretory syndrome. Non-functioning NETs are indistinguishable from RCC metastases; thus, in such patients only a history of nephrectomy can lead to the correct diagnosis. Also helpful is that metastatic lesions are typically multi-focal (Fig. 15.4) at the time of diagnosis. Consequently, to obtain a final diagnosis, biopsy must be accompanied by panoramic imaging studies for tumor staging.

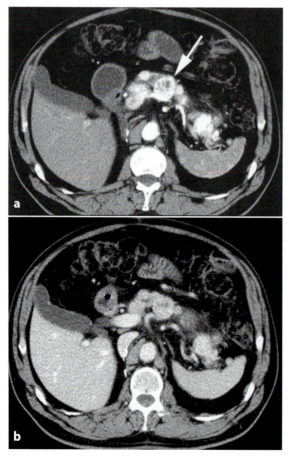

Fig. 15.4 CT scan showing metastastic renal cell carcinoma (RCC) to the pancreas. Multiple nodules (*arrow*) in the pancreatic gland are characteristically hypervascular in the arterial phase (**a**) and vascularized also in the venous phase (**b**)

The imaging methods most often used in clinical practice, including for the detection of metastatic RCC, is multi-detector computed tomography (MDCT) due to its high spatial and temporal resolution, which allows the identification of small lesions. As noted above, pancreatic metastasis of RCC are usually hypervascular, which makes them readily detectable in the arterial phase of a contrast-enhanced MDCT examination (Fig. 15.4a). Sometimes, in larger lesions, hypodense central areas of necrosis are present. In later phases of the contrast-enhanced MDCT study, the lesions may be more difficult to detect because the difference in the density of the mass vs. that of the normal pancreatic gland decreases (Fig. 15.4b). Other rare and non-specific features of these lesions are calcifications, ductal and biliary obstruction, vascular extension, and cystic degeneration.

15.3.3 Treatment

Surgical Treatment for Resectable Disease
The first report of a pancreatic resection for metastatic RCC was published 60 years ago [26]. Since then, results have been published as case reports, small single-institution series, and, more recently, as in-depth reviews of the entire literature [12, 13, 19, 27].

Since RCC metastases to the pancreas are rare, prospective randomized trials to evaluate the role of surgical resection in the multi-modal treatment of these patients have not been possible. In fact, there have been no more than 500 reported pancreatic resections over these last 60 years, and the conclusions are not sufficiently definitive to comprise an adequate level of evidence. Furthermore, only a few authors have tried to compare outcomes in patients with resected and non-resected disease [13, 19, 28], with debatable results due to the difficulty of the comparisons. For example, among the latter group, single pancreatic metastases are rare and diffuse extrapancreatic disease at the time of the diagnosis is frequently observed [28].

Despite these intrinsic limitations, some evidence is available to guide therapeutic decision-making in patients with RCC pancreatic metastasis. Firstly, accurate staging, including a total-body CT scan, is necessary to discover asymptomatic distant metastases to the brain and lung, while bone scintigraphy should be performed to exclude skeletal metastases. Another tool useful in the risk stratification of these patients, developed to ensure that only those who will truly benefit from surgical resection will be offered this form of treatment, was recently developed at the Memorial Sloan Kettering Cancer Center (MSKCC) [29]. This prognostic model divides patients into one of three classes based upon five parameters: time to recurrence (< or > 12 months), tumor burden (LDH), hematopoietic suppression or skeletal involvement (serum hemoglobin and calcium), and performance status. A final score of 0 points identifies a group considered to be at favorable risk: metachronous metastasis arising > 1 year after nephrectomy, serum hemoglobin > 13 and

11.5 gm/dl in males and females, respectively, serum calcium < 10 mg/dl, serum LDH < 300 U/l, and Karnofsky performance status ≥ 80%. Intermediate risk patients have a score of 1–2 points and those at high risk a score of 3–5 points. If extrapancreatic disease has been ruled out, most authors agree that a surgical approach to the lesion should be recommended whenever a R0 resection is likely to be achieved in a favorable risk patient.

The surgical technique should be based on a well-defined protocol, similar to that developed for pancreatic NETs in MEN1 patients. In fact, RCC metastases in the pancreas are multiple in up to 45% of surgical specimens, as widely reported in the recent literature [13, 19, 28, 30], but multiple nodules are well documented in the preoperative diagnostic work-up only in half of the pathological cases [28, 30]. Following accurate palpation of the entire gland after its wide exposure along its posterior surface, intraoperative US (IOUS) should be performed for lesion detection and to allow a surgical resection with a minimally invasive approach. IOUS provides details on the contiguity between the lesions and the main pancreatic duct, enabling the surgeon to choose the most appropriate approach to the nodule. Whenever possible, any single nodule is preferably resected while sparing healthy parenchyma, thus avoiding a total pancreatectomy. However, the latter is mandatory if the multiple nodules are large and involve the main pancreatic duct. In case of body and tail lesions and a small nodule in the uncinate process that does not involve the Wirsung duct, a distal pancreatectomy associated with an enucleation of the main nodule is warranted. Frozen sections of the resected margins are mandatory. An initial report of a high local recurrence rate after parenchyma-sparing surgery [30] was not confirmed in subsequent reports. Nonetheless, the entire gland should be carefully inspected in order to detect any single lesion [28, 31], avoiding removal of the pancreas due to a fear of local relapse. Indeed, despite the adoption of a policy of atypical resection [28, 31], the incidence of pancreatic recurrences was negligible. An adequate follow-up with US or magnetic resonance imaging (MRI) is strongly encouraged given the possibility of a new localization in the remnant pancreas, which occurs in 4% of cases according to a recent complete literature review [19], but also because of the high rate (17%) of extrapancreatic recurrences after pancreatic resection. However, new localizations of RCC are still amenable to surgical resection, as the disease can eventually be eradicated in around 45% of patients]19]. Standard peri-pancreatic lymph node dissection is largely sufficient because the rate of nodal involvement is negligible in most series, with an incidence of 10% reported by the Johns Hopkins Surgical Department [32] and 20% by the Heidelberg Surgical Department [31]; the latter is the highest ever reported.

Some authors have suggested performing multi-visceral resections in patients whose pancreatic metastases are associated with extrapancreatic disease [19, 31]. Based on the consistent postoperative morbidity and mortality of these patients and the substantial worsening of the prognosis, the recommendation is a multi-disciplinary evaluation, including the oncologist, of such cases. If surgery is not necessary to palliate symptoms, it is probably better to initially observe the patients and administer systemic treatment [19]. A new staging of patients with multi-metastatic disease can then identify those who presumably have a better chance of benefit from a multi-visceral surgical resection.

Even though the metastases may be confined to the pancreas, they may not be resectable because they have infiltrated the superior mesenteric axis, in particular the superior mesenteric artery or the celiac trunk. The final diagnosis can be easily reached by US-guided percutaneous FNA [33]. Whenever symptoms such as duodenal obstruction or jaundice are present, a palliative procedure is indicated because of the relatively good prognosis of patients with non-resectable metastases [19].

Medical Treatment for Non-resectable Disease

Patients with stage IV RCC with synchronous or metachronous initially non-resectable solitary pancreatic metastases, or with multiple metastatic sites including the pancreas that are not amenable to surgery should be offered systemic therapy.

In the past, systemic treatment options for metastatic RCC were limited to various combinations and dosages of interleukin (IL)-2 and interferon (IFN). In most of cases, the clinical benefit to the patients was limited and treatment was burdened by significant toxicities.

More recently, based on important advances in our knowledge of the molecular mechanisms involved in the progression of this disease, several targeted agents have been developed and approved for the first and second-line treatment of advanced RCC, including sunitinib, sorafenib, pazopanib, temsirolimus, everolimus, and bevacizumab in combination with IFN. Tumor histology and risk assessment are the main criteria in the selection of patients for targeted therapies.

Sunitinib is a multi-kinase inhibitor targeting different tyrosine kinase receptors, including platelet-derived growth factor receptors (PDGFR-a and -b), vascular endothelial growth factor receptors (VEGFR-1, -2, and -3), stem cell factor receptor (c-KIT), FMS-like tyrosine kinase (FLT-3), colony-stimulating factor (CSF-1R), and neurotrophic factor receptor (RET) [34, 35]. Sunitinib has been recently approved as first-line treatment of unresectable RCC, based on the positive results of a large phase III trial in which 750 previously untreated patients with metastatic RCC were randomly assigned to receive either sunitinib or IFN [34]. Although most of the patients selected for the trial had clear cell RCCs of either "favorable" or "intermediate" MSKCC risk, recent data from an expanded access trial revealed that sunitinib has an acceptable safety profile and activity also in subgroups of patients with non-clear-cell histology tumors, brain metastases, and poor performance status [36].

A second, pharmacologically relevant target in RCC is the mammalian target of rapamycin (mTOR) protein, a serine/threonine protein kinase that regulates cell growth, proliferation, and survival in the context of different multiprotein mTOR complexes, referred to as mTORC1 and mTORC2. Temsirolimus is an inhibitor of mTOR and is recommended for the first-line treatment of relapsed or unresectable clear-cell stage IV RCC in patients who therefore have a poor prognosis. The efficacy and safety of temsirolimus were demonstrated in a phase III study in which untreated patients with advanced RCC who had three or more of six unfavorable prognostic factors were randomized to receive temsirolimus, IFN, or both [37]. The group of patients who received temsirolimus alone showed a significant improvement in overall survival compared to those receiving IFN alone or both drugs.

Several targeted agents have been also approved as subsequent therapy in patients with tumors having a predominantly clear-cell histology. Everolimus is an orally available mTOR inhibitor approved for use in patients after failure of treatment with tyrosine kinase inhibitors [38]. Axitinib is a selective, second-generation inhibitor of VEGFR 1–3, approved for the treatment of patients with advanced RCC after failure of one prior systemic therapy [39], including sunitinib, bevacizumab plus IFN, temsirolimus, or cytokines [40].

15.3.4 Pathology

Renal cell carcinoma tends to metastasize as a solitary mass but can also result in multiple lesions. Grossly metastatic RCC presents as a well-circumscribed yellow-orange tumor with red-brown or white-gray areas (Fig. 15.5) and can show hemorrhagic or cystic degeneration (Fig. 15.6). Clear-cell RCC is the most common histologic type that metastasizes to the pancreas.

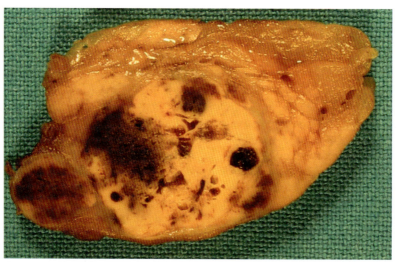

Fig. 15.5 Gross appearance of metastatic RCC: well-circumscribed yellow-orange to red-brown mass

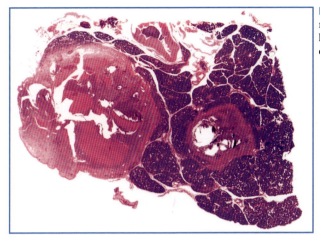

Fig. 15.6 Two nodules of metastatic RCC, with hemorrhage and cystic degeneration

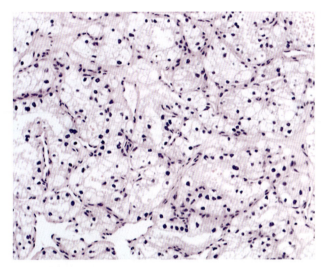

Fig. 15.7 Metastatic RCC: sheets, small nests, and cords of clear cells separated by a rich sinusoidal vascular network

Microscopically, metastatic clear-cell RCC is a cell-rich tumor organized in sheets, small nests, or cords of polygonal clear cells (Fig. 15.7). These cells have abundant clear, cytoplasm because of the accumulation of glycogen, which can be easily demonstrated with PAS. Metastatic clear-cell RCCs are highly vascularized. At imaging, the main differential diagnosis is pancreatic NETs. In such cases, immunohistochemistry is a worthwhile diagnostic tool because metastatic RCC shows typical reactivity for CD10 and CD13, but it is negative for endocrine markers such as chromogranin and synaptophysin.

15.3.5 Prognostic Factors

Overall survival for isolated solitary or multiple RCC pancreatic metastases was 57% in an extensive review [17] and up to 88% [28] in a single-center series.

The prognosis of patients with RCC pancreatic metastases depends on a limited number of factors. Patients who present with multi-organ metastases associated with pancreatic metastases have the poorest prognosis. In this subset, an R0 resection often cannot be achieved; the 2- and 5- year overall survival rates were 41% and 14%, respectively, in historical series [19]. These patients are candidates for medical treatment with bevacizumab, sorafenib, tensirolimus, and sunitinib. If all the metastases are resected together with the involved pancreas, extrapancreatic disease is the only significant prognostic factor for disease-free survival [19].

It is widely recognized that the longer the interval between nephrectomy and metastases, the better the outcome of the patient, with a cut-off ranging between 2 and 3 years of latency. However, a previous history of a solitary RCC metastasis at extrapancreatic sites should not be considered a contraindication to pancreatic resection [19, 31]. Also, the usual multiplicity and the size of the metastases do not alter disease-free and overall survival after complete excision. Only Reddy [32]. reported lymph node involvement as a prognostic factor in addition to vascular invasion, but these data have to be considered with prudence because they represent an isolated experience involving only a few patients.

References

1. Rock J, Bloomston M, Lozanski G, Frankel WL (2012) The spectrum of hematologic malignancies involving the pancreas: potential clinical mimics of pancreatic adenocarcinoma. Am J Clin Pathol 37:414-422
2. Adsay NV, Andrea A, Basturk O et al (2004) Secondary tumors of the pancreas: an analysis of a surgical and autopsy database and review of the literature. Virchows Arch 444:527-535
3. Sweeney AD, Fisher WE, Wu MF et al (2010) Value of Pancreatic Resection for Cancer Metastatic to the Pancreas, J Surg Res 160:268-276
4. Washington K, McDonagh D (1994) Secondary tumors of the gastrointestinal tract: surgical pathologic findings and comparison with autopsy survey. Mod Pathol 8:427-433
5. Z'graggen K, Fernandez-del Castillo C, Rattner DW et al (1998) Metastases to the pancreas and their surgical extirpation. Arch Surg 133:413-418
6. Robbins EG II, Franceschi D, Barkin JS (1996) Solitary metastatic tumors to the pancreas: a case report and a review of the literature. Am J Gastroenterol 91:2414-2417
7. Konstantinidis IT, Dursun A, Zheng H (2010) Metastatic tumors in the pancreas in the modern era. J Am Coll Surg 211:749-753
8. Moutardier V, Berthet B, Le Treut Y (1993) Metastase pancreatique d'une tumeur de Grawitz. J Chir (Paris) 130:439-440
9. Altschuler EL, Ray A (1998) Spontaneous regression of a pancreatic metastasis of a renal cell carcinoma. Arch Fam Med 7:516-517

10. Motzer RJ, Bander NH, Nanus DM (1996) Renal-cell carcinoma. N Engl J Med 335:865-875
11. Reddy S, Wolfgang CI (2009) The role of surgery in the management of isolated metastases to the pancreas. Lancet Oncol 10:287-293
12. Kassabian A, Stein J, Jabbour N (2000) Renal cell carcinoma metastatic to the pancreas: a single-institution series and review of the literature. Urology 56:211-215
13. Sellner F, Tykalsky N, De Santis M et al (2006) Solitary and multiple isolated metastases of clear cell renal carcinoma to the pancreas: an indication for pancreatic surgery. Ann Surg Oncol 13:75-85
14. Ward Y, Wang W, Woodhouse E et al (2001) Signal pathways which promote invasion and metastasis: critical and distinct contributions of extra-cellular signal-regulated kinase and Ral-specific guanine exchange factor pathways. Mol Cell Biol 21:5958-5969
15. Hiotis SP, Klimstra DS, Conlon KC, Brennan MF (2002) Results after pancreatic resection for metastatic lesions. Ann Surg Oncol 9:675-679
16. Le Borgne J, Partensky C, Glemain P et al (2000) Pancreaticoduodenectomy for metastatic ampullary and pancreatic tumors. Hepatogastroenterology 47:540-544
17. Thompson LD, Heffess CS et al (2000) Renal cell carcinoma to the pancreas in surgical pathology material. Cancer 89:1076-1088
18. Fabre JM, Rouanet P, Dagues F et al (1995) Various features and surgical approach of solitary pancreatic metastasis from renal cell carcinoma. Eur J Surg Oncol 21:683-686
19. Tanis PJ, van der Gaag NA, Busch OR et al (2009) Systematic review of pancreatic surgery for metastatic renal cell carcinoma. Br J Surg 96:579-592
20. Faure JP, Tuech JJ, Richer JP et al (2001) Pancreatic metastasis of renal cell carcinoma: presentation, treatment and survival. J Urol 165:20-22
21. Law CH, Wei AC, Hanna SS et al (2003) Pancreatic resection for metastatic renal cell carcinoma: presentation, treatment, and outcome. Ann Surg Oncol 10:922-926
22. Sohn TA, Yeo CJ, Cameron JL et al (2001) Renal cell carcinoma metastatic to the pancreas: results of surgical management. J Gastrointest Surg 5:346-351
23. Mechó S, Quiroga S, Cuéllar H, Sebastià C (2009) Pancreatic metastasis of renal cell carcinoma: multidetector CT findings. Abdom Imaging 34:385-389
24. Flath B, Rickes S, Schweigert M et al (2003) Differentiation of pancreatic metastasis of a renal cell carcinoma from primary pancreatic carcinoma by echo-enhanced power Doppler sonography. Pancreatology 3:349-351
25. Megibow AJ (2003) Secondary pancreatic tumors: imaging. In: Procacci C, Megibow AJ (eds) Imaging of the pancreas. Cystic and rare tumors. Springer-Verlag: Berlin, pp 277-288.
26. Jenssen E (1952) A metastatic hypernephroma to the pancreas. Acta Chir Scand 104:177-180
27. Ballarin R, Spaggiari M, Cautero N et al (2011) Pancreatic metastases from renal cell carcinoma: the state of the art. World J Gastroenterol 17:4747-4756
28. Zerbi A, Ortolano E, Balzano G et al (2008) Pancreatic metastasis from renal cell carcinoma: which patients benefit from surgical resection? Ann Surg Oncol 15:1161-1168
29. Motzer JR, Mazumdar M, Bacik J et al (1999) Survival and prognostic stratification of 670 patients with advanced renal cell carcinoma. J Clin Oncol 17:2530-2540
30. Bassi C, Butturini G, Falconi M et al (2003) High recurrence rate after atypical resection for pancreatic metastases from renal cell carcinoma. Br J Surg 90:555-559
31. Strobel O, Hackert T, Hartwig W et al (2009) Survival data justifies resection for pancreatic metastases. Ann Surg Oncol 16:3340-3349
32. Reddy S, Edil BH, Cameron JL et al (2008) Pancreatic resection of isolated metastases from nonpancreatic primary cancers. Ann Surg Oncol 15:3199-3206
33. Butturini G, Bassi C, Falconi M et al (1998) Surgical treatment of pancreatic metastases from renal cell carcinomas. Dig Surg 15:241-246
34. Motzer RJ, Hutson TE, Tomczak P et al (2007) Sunitinib versus interferon alfa in metastatic renal-cell carcinoma. N Engl J Med 356:115-124
35. Motzer RJ, Michaelson MD, Redman BG et al (2006) Activity of SU11248, a multitargeted inhibitor of vascular endothelial growth factor receptor and platelet-derived growth factor receptor, in patients with metastatic renal cell carcinoma. J Clin Oncol 24:16-24

36. Gore ME, Szczylik C, Porta C et al (2009) Safety and efficacy of sunitinib for metastatic renal-cell carcinoma: an expanded-access trial. Lancet Oncol 10:757-763
37. Hudes G, Carducci M, Tomczak P et al (2007) Temsirolimus, interferon alfa, or both for advanced renal-cell carcinoma. N Engl J Med 356:2271-2281
38. Motzer RJ, Escudier B, Oudard S et al (2008) Efficacy of everolimus in advanced renal cell carcinoma: a double-blind, randomised, placebo-controlled phase III trial. Lancet 372:449-456
39. Sonpavde G, Hutson TE, Rini BI (2008) Axitinib for renal cell carcinoma. Expert Opin Investig Drugs 17:741-748
40. Rini BI, Escudier B, Tomczak P et al (2011) Comparative effectiveness of axitinib versus sorafenib in advanced renal cell carcinoma (AXIS): a randomised phase 3 trial. Lancet 378:1931-1939

Primary Non-epithelial Tumors of the Pancreas

16

Marco Dal Molin and Paola Capelli

16.1 Introduction

Primary non-epithelial tumors of the pancreas are exceedingly rare. By contrast, those arising from neighboring sites, especially gastrointestinal stromal tumors and sarcomas arising from the retroperitoneum, may secondarily involve the pancreatic gland. There is also a wide range of benign mesenchymal tumors, including vascular tumors, fibromatosis (solid desmoid tumor), solitary fibrous tumors, schwannomas, and several others that can involve the pancreas. Some primary sarcomas have also been shown to have a pancreatic localization. The histologic features of these neoplasms are thus highly variable, as they include tumors of vascular origin, primitive neuroectodermal tumors, synovial sarcomas, desmoplastic small round-cell tumors [1], leiomyosarcomas, malignant fibrous histiocytomas, and others.

In this chapter, we review the broad spectrum of primary mesenchymal tumors that may involve the pancreas, most of which are largely documented in single case reports. In addition, we focus on their pathologic features, as well as their current diagnostic and therapeutic management.

16.2 Benign Mesenchymal Tumors

A large variety of benign soft-tissue neoplasms has been described in the pancreas, including several types of vascular tumors, such as hemangioendothelioma [2, 3], cavernous hemangioma [4], and hemangioma not otherwise defined [5, 6].

M. Dal Molin (✉)
Department of Surgery and Oncology, General Surgery Unit, Pancreas Center,
"G.B. Rossi" University Hospital,
Verona, Italy
e-mail: marcodalmo82@gmail.com

P. Pederzoli and C. Bassi (eds.), *Uncommon Pancreatic Neoplasms*,
Updates in Surgery
DOI: 10.1007/978-88-470-2673-5_16, © Springer-Verlag Italia 2013

Pancreatic lymphangioma [7, 8] and cystic lymphangioma [9-11] are rare. These multicystic tumors are 3–20 cm in diameter and characterized by serous or chylous fluid-filled cystic spaces. The stroma may contain smooth muscle cells and lymphocytes. Abdominal lymphangioma has also been reported to mimic a pancreatic cystic neoplasm [12], while an infiltrating cavernous lymphangiomyoma can involve the pancreas secondarily [13].

Given its rich innervation [14], it is not surprising that neural tumors can arise from the pancreas; examples of such neoplasms are schwannoma [15] and neurofibroma [16]. Based on a recent review, the largest available to date, 37 cases of primary pancreatic schwannoma have been reported in total [17].

The diagnostic work-up of this class of tumors is based on standard imaging techniques, including computed tomography (CT) and abdominal magnetic resonance imaging (MRI) studies. However, the radiologic aspect is not specific and tumor markers are usually negative, such that histological analysis of the surgical specimen is therefore required to obtain the diagnosis. When resection is radical, surgical treatment is usually curative.

Several cases of pancreatic paraganglioma have been reported in the literature [18]. These are rare neuroendocrine neoplasms (NENs) arising in the extra-adrenal chromaffin cells of the autonomic nervous system. Although seldom, para-gangliomas can occur around and involve the pancreas, thereby mimicking one of the more common primary pancreatic tumors. In a series of nine peri-pancreatic para-gangliomas recently described [19], patients either presented clinically with diffuse epigastric and abdominal pain or an incidental mass was discovered on routine radiographic imaging. In all patients these masses were suspected as being a primary pancreatic neoplasm on radiographic examination, were predominantly located in the body of the pancreas, and ranged in size from 5.5 to 17.0 cm in diameter. If the nature of the tumor is not suspected based on other information, then interpretation of the fine-needle aspiration (FNA) biopsy and even the pathology examination of the surgical specimens can be challenging. Close follow-up of these patients should be considered because of the significant risk of metastatic disease.

16.3   Malignant Mesenchymal Tumors

Primary malignant sarcomas of the pancreas are rare neoplasms that display a wide range of histological features. The prognosis of patients with pancreatic mesenchymal tumors parallels that of patients with sarcomas arising in other sites. Within this group of neoplasms, leiomyosarcoma represents the most frequent entity [20] (Fig. 16.1), followed by malignant fibrous histiocytoma [21], fibrosarcoma [22], liposarcoma [23], and malignant peripheral nerve sheath tumor [24]. In exceedingly rare conditions, malignant sarcomas arising in the extremities or in the retroperitoneum can metastasize to other organs, including the pancreas. The first case of pleomorphic liposarcoma metastasizing to the pancreas was recently described in a 30-year-old-man,

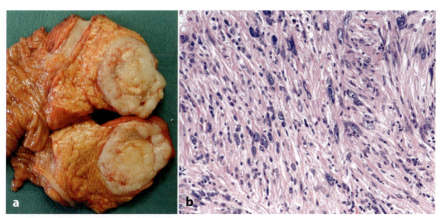

Fig. 16.1 Metastatic leioomyosarcoma. **a** Gross appearance of a mesenchymal tumor: the tumor is well circumscribed and composed of soft tissue. **b** Histologically, the tumor exhibits high cellularity and is composed of spindle cells with atypia

who underwent distal pancreatectomy with splenectomy [25].

Based on a review of the current literature, only 29 cases of primary pancreatic leiomyosarcomas have been reported [26]. These tumors can range from 1.0 to 30.0 cm in diameter, with an equal distribution among men and women. Symptoms are usually present at the time of diagnosis; although none of these are specific, patients may complain of abdominal pain, jaundice, and weight loss. Aggressive surgical treatment is usually advocated, as these neoplasms respond poorly to systemic treatments. Pancreatic leiomyosarcomas tend to metastasize to other organs, especially the liver whereas lymph node metastases are unusual.

References

1. Bismar TA, Basturk O, Gerald WL (2004) Desmoplastic small cell tumor in the pancreas. Am J Surg Pathol 28:808-812
2. Chappell JS (1973) Case reports. Benign hemangioendothelioma of the head of the pancreas treated by pancreaticoduodenectomy. J Pediatr Surg 8:431-432
3. Tunell WP (1976) Hemangioendothelioma of the pancreas obstructing the common bile duct and duodenum. J Pediatr Surg 11:827-830
4. Mundinger GS, Gust S, Micchelli ST et al (2009) Adult pancreatic hemangioma: case report and literature review. Gastroenterol Res Pract 2009:839730
5. Lee J, Raman K, Sachithanandan S (2011) Pancreatic hemangioma mimicking a malignant pancreatic cyst. Gastrointest Endosc 73:174-176
6. Künzli BM, Shrikhande SV, Büchler MW, Friess H (2004) Pancreatic lesions in von Hippel-Lindau syndrome: report of a case. Surg Today 34:626-629
7. Epstein HS, Berman R (1975) Mesenteric and pancreatic lymphangioma presenting as a right adnexal mass. Am J Obstet Gynecol 121:1117-1118
8. Paal E, Thompson LD, Heffess CS (1998) A clinicopathologic and immunohistochemical study of ten pancreatic lymphangiomas and a review of the literature. Cancer 82:2150-2158

9. Fahimi H, Faridi M, Gholamin S et al (2010) Cystic lymphangioma of the pancreas: diagnostic and therapeutic challenges. JOP 11:617-619
10. Navina S, Kaplan KJ (2009) Cystic lymphangioma of the pancreas. ANZ J Surg 79:409
11. Colovic RB, Grubor NM, Micev MT et al (2008) Cystic lymphangioma of the pancreas. World J Gastroenterol 14:6873-6875
12. Khandelwal M, Lichtenstein GR, Morris JB et al (1995) Abdominal lymphangioma masquerading as a pancreatic cystic neoplasm. J Clin Gastroenterol 20:142-144
13. Iqbal J, Isaacs P, Sissons M et al (2009) A cause for concern? An asymptomatic mesenteric lesion. Cavernous lymphangioma Gut 58:1184-1225
14. Mössner J (2010) New advances in cell physiology and pathophysiology of the exocrine pancreas. Dig Dis 28:722-728
15. Suzuki S, Kaji S, Koike N et al (2010) Pancreatic schwannoma: a case report and literature review with special reference to imaging features. JOP 11:31-35
16. Kato O, Hattori K, Matsuyama M, Yoshizaki S (1982) Neurofibroma of the pancreas: differentiation from carcinoma. Am J Gastroenterol 77:630-632
17. Gupta A, Subhas G, Mittal VK, Jacobs MJ (2009) Pancreatic schwannoma: literature review. J Surg Educ 66:168-173
18. Vermeulen BJ, Widgren S, Gur V et al (1990) Dermoid cyst of the pancreas. Case report and review of the literature. Gastroenterol Clin Biol 14:1023-1025
19. Cope C, Greenberg SH, Vidal JJ, Cohen EA (1974) Nonfunctioning nonchromaffin paraganglioma of the pancreas. Arch Surg 109:440-442
20. Zhang H, Jensen MH, Farnell MB et al (2010) Primary leiomyosarcoma of the pancreas: study of 9 cases and review of literature. Am J Surg Pathol 34:1849-1856
21. Allen KB, Skandalakis LJ, Brown BC et al (1990) Malignant fibrous histiocytoma of the pancreas. Am Surg 56:364-368
22. Brooke WS, Maxwell JG (1966) Primary sarcoma of the pancreas. Eight year survival after pancreatoduodenectomy. Am J Surg 112:657-661
23. Elliott TE, Albertazzi VJ, Danto LA (1980) Pancreatic liposarcoma: case report with review of retroperitoneal liposarcomas. Cancer 45:1720-1723
24. Hirose T, Maeda T, Furuya K et al (1998) Malignant peripheral nerve sheath tumor of the pancreas with perineurial cell differentiation. Ultrastruct Pathol 22:227-231
25. Malleo G, Crippa S, Partelli S et al (2009) Pleomorphic liposarcoma of the axilla metastatic to the pancreas. Dig Surg 26:262-263
26. Zhang H, Jensen MH, Farnell MB et al (2010) Primary leiomyosarcoma of the pancreas: study of 9 cases and review of literature. Am J Surg Pathol 34:1849-1856

Tumor-like Lesions of the Pancreas

17

Luca Frulloni, Antonio Amodio, Italo Vantini,
Marco Dal Molin, Marco Inama, Mirko D'Onofrio,
Lisa Marcolini, Claudio Luchini, Giovanni Butturini
and Paola Capelli

17.1 Autoimmune Pancreatitis

Autoimmune pancreatitis (AIP) is a "one of a kind" inflammatory disease of the pancreas since it differs clinically, pathologically, and instrumentally from all other types of pancreatitis. Many papers have been published since the introduction of the term "autoimmune pancreatitis" by Yoshida et al. in 1995 [1], focusing mainly on the dramatic and quick response to steroid therapy.

AIP has been recently classified as *type 1* (also called lymphoplasmacytic sclerosing pancreatitis, LPSP) and *type 2* (idiopathic duct centric pancreatitis, *IDCP*) [2]. Type 1 AIP is characterized by the presence of storiform fibrosis, with obstructive phlebitis (Fig. 17.1); high levels of serum IgG4; and IgG4+ plasma cells in the involved pancreatic tissue. Other pathologic findings may be observed in this form of AIP, but they are not specific and are shared with type 2 AIP (Fig. 17.2). Type 2 AIP is characterized mainly by the presence of *granulocytic epithelial lesions* (GEL), which are the expression of an aggressive cellular attack against the pancreatic epithelial ductal cells, with rupture and destruction of ductal structures [3].

The clinical profiles of patients suffering from AIP seems to differ in the two forms of the disease [4]. Patients with type 1 AIP are older, with a higher prevalence of males and a more frequent involvement of other organs, both of the gastrointestinal tract and extra-gastrointestinal. The main clinical implication of this classification seems to be that type 1 AIP is a systemic relapsing IgG4-associated disease, whereas type 2 AIP is a serum IgG4-negative disease that does not relapse. However, the frequency of relapse(s) seems to

---

L. Frulloni (✉)
Department of Medicine, Pancreas Center, "G.B. Rossi" University Hospital,
Verona, Italy
e-mail: luca.frulloni@univr.it

P. Pederzoli and C. Bassi (eds.), *Uncommon Pancreatic Neoplasms*,
Updates in Surgery
DOI: 10.1007/978-88-470-2673-5_16, © Springer-Verlag Italia 2013

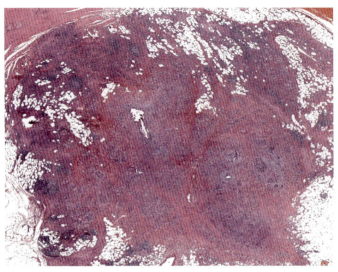

Fig. 17.1 Autoimmune pancreatitis Whole-mount section of the head of the pancreas: ill-defined, firm mass extending into the peri-pancreatic tissues and narrowing the secondary ducts

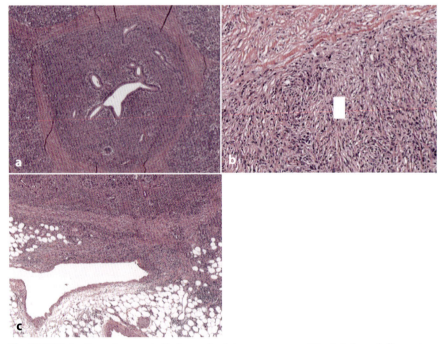

Fig. 17.2 Distinctive microscopic findings of autoimmune pancreatitis. **a** A dense inflammatory infiltrate is centered on medium-sized to large pancreatic duct. **b** Storiform pattern of fibrosis. **c** Obliterative venulitis: the inflammatory cells infiltrate a venous wall

be similar in the two forms of AIP, according to a recent paper from a French series [5].

AIP is a disease that quickly and fully responds to steroids [6-9]. The initial dosage of prednisolone ranges from 0.5 to 1 mg/kg/day, tapering to 2.5–5 mg every week.

The concept of the disease has changed over the time. Initially, AIP was considered to involve the entire pancreas, based on the Japanese experience. Later, the possibility of a segmental inflammatory involvement of the pancreas was proposed. Therefore, a clinically based classification of *focal* vs. *diffuse* AIP is now generally accepted [7, 10]. Focal AIP is defined as a segmental involvement of the pancreatic parenchyma with or without the presence of a low-density mass, as determined at imaging. In an Italian series, focal AIP was more frequent than diffuse AIP (63% vs. 37%) [7]. Compared to diffuse AIP, patients with focal AIP are older, more frequently males, and the main clinical presentation is jaundice. Since these findings are shared with pancreatic cancer, many patients with AIP undergo resective surgery (pancreaticoduodenectomy).

Indeed, this morphologically based classification has important clinical implications since in the presence of a focal disease, particularly if a low-density mass is detected at imaging, pancreatic cancer must be carefully and confidently excluded before steroid therapy is introduced [11]. The risk is, on the one hand, to operate on a patient with AIP that fully responds to steroids and, on the other, to treat a resectable cancer with steroids, delaying surgery and exposing the patient to the possibility of metastases or local invasion, both of which may preclude surgery. The diagnostic algorithm is therefore different in focal and diffuse forms of AIP.

In diffuse forms, a cholangiocarcinoma may be suspected in the presence of a single stenosis of the common bile duct. However, the probability of this being a malignancy (cholangiocarcinoma, peri-ampullar neoplasia) is very low and the differential diagnosis should mainly include acute pancreatitis (Figs. 17.3, 17.4).

By contrast, in the focal forms the likelihood of a cancer is very high. A recent review of the studies investigating the frequency of benign disease in patients who underwent pancreatic surgery for a resectable mass in the head of the pancreas found that 10% of these patients had an inflammatory pancreatic disease [11]. A recent study reported that half of these patients had a final diagnosis of LPSP. Therefore, in the presence of a pancreatic mass, only one patient in ten can be expected to have an inflammatory disease, while the large majority have a malignancy. The implication for clinical practice is that in the presence of a pancreatic mass pancreatic cancer needs to be excluded before patients are treated with steroids. Despite radiological, serological, and clinical findings highly suggestive of AIP, we strongly recommend that a biopsy of the pancreas be performed in such cases. For this purpose, fine-needle aspiration (FNA) biopsy is more accurate than core biopsy in the exclusion of cancer. Figure 17.5 shows the algorithm we propose in focal AIP with or without

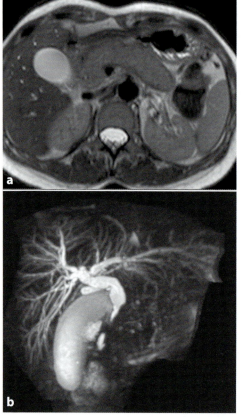

Fig. 17.3 MRI findings of a patient suffering from the diffuse form of autoimmune pancreatitis. **a** The axial sequence shows a diffuse enlargement of the pancreas, with a peripheral rim. **b** MRCP shows a stenosis of the intrapancreatic segment of the common bile duct with upstream dilation of the extra- and intrahepatic trees, without dilation of the main pancreatic duct

a hypodense mass at imaging. A trial with high-dose steroid therapy (1 mg/kg/day) may lead to a definitive diagnosis of AIP and should be made only if cytology is negative and the results of imaging, i.e., CT (Fig. 17.6), magnetic resonance imaging (MRI), endoscopic ultrasound (EUS), or contrast-enhanced EUS, are suggestive of AIP. At an international meeting held in Fukuoka, Japan, international consensus diagnostic criteria (ICDC) were recently proposed and can be used in this setting [12] (Figs. 17.5, 17.7). A second look after 3 weeks with the same imaging technique used at the basal examination is required. Normalization or significant improvement of the pancreatic morphology (disappearance of the hypodense mass, normalization of the pancreatic ductal system) is an important diagnostic finding. However, the decision to use steroids is difficult and should be made in an experienced tertiary center, after discussions among clinicians, radiologists, and surgeons.

17 Tumor-like Lesions of the Pancreas

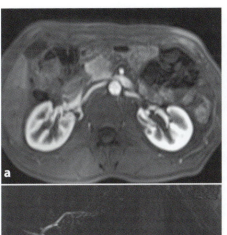

Fig. 17.4 MRI findings of a patient suffering from the focal form of autoimmune pancreatitis. **a** The axial sequence shows focal involvement in the head of the pancreas, with a hypodense mass mimicking a pancreatic adenocarcinoma. **b** MRCP demonstrates a stenosis of the intrapancreatic segment of the common bile duct, with upstream mild dilation of the extra- and intrahepatic trees, and a long stenosis of the main pancreatic duct in the head of the pancreas

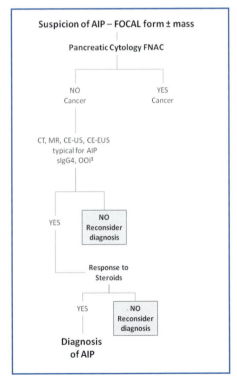

Fig. 17.5 Diagnostic algorithm for patients with the focal form of autoimmune pancreatitis according to the ICDC for AIP [12]

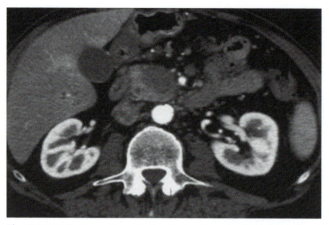

Fig. 17.6 CT findings of a patient suffering from the focal form of autoimmune pancreatitis

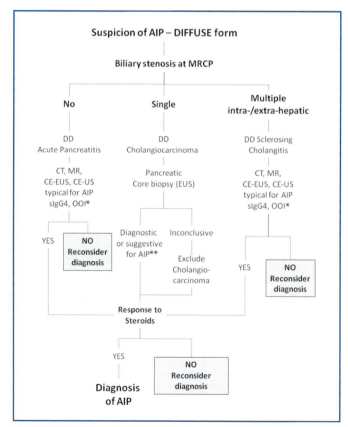

Fig. 17.7 Diagnostic algorithm for patients with the diffuse form of autoimmune pancreatitis, using the international consensus diagnostic criteria (ICDC) for AIP [12] (*) or the criteria of Zamboni et al. [3] (**)

17.2 Paraduodenal Pancreatitis

17.2.1 Epidemiology, Etiology and Pathogenesis

Chronic pancreatitis (CP) reflects a chronic inflammatory process involving the pancreas, with a final result of endocrine and exocrine pancreatic insufficiency. Reports of the prevalence of CP vary enormously, from 20 to 200 cases per 100,000 people described in the general population, with the increase due to the rising consumption of alcohol [13]. CP has a very long course and the involvement of the duodenal wall is typical; stenosis occurs in 19.6–31% of all cases of CP [14, 15]. The duodenal wall can be affected by other rare conditions, such as enterogenous duplication and retention cysts of the Brunner glands, or as a result of pancreatitis in duodenal heterotopic pancreas. The latter has been described under different names (para-ampullary duodenal wall cyst, cystic dystrophy of the duodenal wall, groove pancreatitis), but considering the clinical presentation along with the radiological and pathological features, we prefer the name paraduodenal pancreatitis (PP) [16]. Typically, PP is seen in male patients in their 40s who have a history of alcohol abuse; the disease involves principally the duodenal wall, near the minor papilla. The pathogenesis of PP has been related to functional and anatomical obstruction of the minor papilla.

Specifically, the minor papilla comprises a ductal system often surrounded by a sphincter-like structure and consistently associated with intraduodenal pancreatic tissue anatomically connected to the dorsocranial pancreas. Therefore, cysts can be considered as dilated ducts associated with intraduodenal pancreas. Of note, intraduodenal pancreatic tissue should be regarded as a bud of the dorsal pancreas entrapped within the duodenal wall during organogenesis, rather than ectopic pancreas. The presence of abundant pancreatic tissue associated with the minor papilla may reflect incomplete migration of the dorsal pancreatic bud and thereby explain the relatively high percentage (67%) of imperforated minor papilla occurring in the normal pancreas. In the presence of a closed minor papilla, countercurrent flow from the duct of Santorini through the duct of Wirsung is generated. It may be impaired by a particularly acute angle of the "Wirsungian knee" [16]. In this scenario, external factors, such as alcohol and smoking, can play a central role, rendering the pancreatic juice more viscous and inducing intrapancreatic calcification. Obstruction of the normal flow of pancreatic juice leads to a chronic inflammatory process and ultimately a paraduodenal mass mimicking a solid-cystic periampullary tumor.

17.2.2 Clinical Presentation and Pathological Features

The clinical presentation of PP reflects the particular location of the pathological process, i.e., the duodenal wall. The most frequent symptom is due to

stenosis of the second duodenal portion, causing pain that is typically amelio-
rated with vomiting. In a minority of patients with PP, the inflammatory
process can involve the "groove" area, compressing the main biliary tract and
thus resulting in jaundice.

Macroscopically, two types of PP may be distinguished. In the "cystic"
type, multiple cysts ranging in diameter from 1 to 10 cm and protruding into
the mucosa of the supra-ampullary duodenum are seen (Fig. 17.8). If the cysts
are particularly large, they may be confused with an intestinal duplication. The
second, "solid" type is characterized by a remarkable thickening of the duodenal wall, which contains cysts less than 1 cm in diameter (Fig. 17.9). Both
types share variable degrees of thickening of the duodenal wall, which is more
evident at the pancreatic side of the second portion of the duodenum, above
the ampulla and connected to the minor papilla. The groove region is usually
enlarged, either due to fibrotic tissue or to the presence of cysts within the
duodenal wall. As a result of the former, narrowing of the common bile duct
may occur, as well as duodenal stenosis secondary to the cysts.

The presence of numerous enlarged peri-pancreatic lymph nodes is also a
typical characteristic of PP.

Histologically, the cysts are found in the submucosal and muscular layers
of the duodenal wall and can often extend to the groove region. Observation
of the cut surface shows that the internal layer of the cysts is mainly lined by
columnar pancreatic ductal cells, which may be lost and replaced by inflammatory granulation tissue. Smooth-muscle hyperplasia and fibrosis, causing
Brunner gland hyperplasia and variable thickening and disarray of the muscular layer in the duodenum, are additional features. The cysts are associated
with heterotopic pancreatic tissue within the muscular or submucosal layer.
More frequently the groove area is characterized by marked fibrosis and
chronic inflammation. Ductal ectasia with stones, fibrosis, and an inflammatory reaction that includes myofibroblastic proliferation are also commonly
observed in the pancreatic parenchyma [17, 18].

17.2.3 Diagnosis and Treatment

In most cases, the clinical and radiological presentations of PP are very similar to those of pancreatic and peri-ampullary tumors, making the differential
diagnosis particularly difficult. The patient's medical history, his or her abuse
of alcohol, weight loss, and the presence of steatorrhea can aid in ruling out
the presence of malignancy. In case of a cystic mass in the groove area, the differential diagnosis is easier, whereas the presence of a solid mass poses a challenge. Imaging can demonstrate the non-specific features that PP shares with
other tumors. Magnetic resonance cholangiopancreatography (MRCP) may
reveal only abnormalities in the biliary and pancreatic ducts. US and contrast-
enhanced CT may show a hypovascularized mass associated with ductal
dilatation and calcification. The identification of small cystic formations in the

17 Tumor-like Lesions of the Pancreas   201

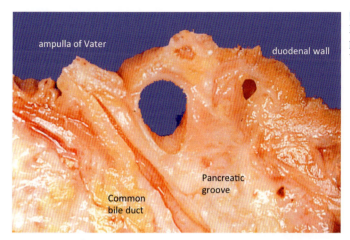

Fig. 17.8
Paraduodenal pancreatitis, cystic variant

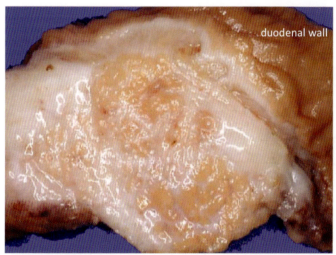

Fig. 17.9
Paraduodenal pancreatitis, solid variant

thickened duodenal wall on the pancreatic side is a specific finding for PP (Fig. 17.10). Procacci et al. [19] described the appearance of the thickened duodenal wall as a solid layer between the duodenal lumen and the pancreas, hypoechoic at US, isoattenuating at unenhanced CT, and hypoattenuating in the early phase and isoattenuating in the late phase on contrast-enhanced CT. The gastroduodenal artery is often dislocated to the left due to the growing mass.

However, the final diagnosis at CT can sometimes be difficult. Consequently, the role of EUS is central in the assessment of solid paraduodenal pancreatic masses. This imaging method is further improved with the use of the newest generation of intravenous contrast agents, but also allows EUS-

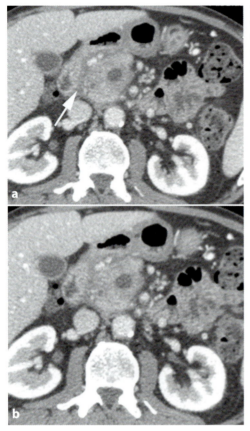

Fig. 17.10 Thickening of the duodenal wall in the groove region, with a hypo-vascularized appearance (*arrow*) at CT (**a, b**). In the pancreatic head, a small pseudocystic lesion is also visible

FNA [20]. The specificity and sensitivity of the latter are between 75–100% and 78–95%, respectively, with a complication rate of 0–2% [21]. EUS-FNA is cost-effective and in our experience is the second most preferred diagnostic method after percutaneous US-guided FNA biopsy.

Surgery represents the best treatment for uncertain pancreatic masses when doubts remain even after EUS-FNA [22]. In this case, surgeons should perform a pancreatoduodenectomy, while the Longmire-Traverso (PD-LT) is the procedure mostly performed for combined obstruction of the duct of Wirsung, main biliary duct, and duodenum [23]. A biliary and duodenal by-pass is indicated in case of duodenal stenosis and jaundice, when endoscopic treatment has failed. In patients with a definitive diagnosis of PP, the immediate elimination of all risks factors (alcohol, smoking) and enzyme replacement are mandatory.

17.3 Pancreatic Hamartoma

Histologically, pancreatic hamartoma is characterized by a focal overgrowth of mature tissue composed of normal cells with a disorderly arrangement [24, 25].

Although these tumors are very rare, their exact prevalence is difficult to determine as some of them are likely to be asymptomatic and remain undetected. In our hospital, a high-volume center for pancreatic pathology, only two cases of pancreatic hamartoma have been collected to date. In both of these, the tumors presented as a solid, well-circumscribed, whitish-gray mass, with a homogeneous appearance on the cut surface and a maximum diameter of 1.5 cm (Fig. 17.11).

Microscopically, pancreatic hamartomas are composed of well-differentiated acinar and ductal cells, without atypia, disposed in a radial trabecular arrangement. A wide sclerotic paucicellular area is usually present in the center of the lesions. Acini and small intralobular and interlobular ducts show atrophic aspects without any evidence of dysplasia. Discrete islets of Langerhans are usually lacking [25] (Fig. 17.12). At preoperative work-up, these lesions are usually misdiagnosed as pancreatic adenocarcinoma; therefore, careful pathological examination is of paramount importance. Of note, repetitive FNA shows normal acinar cells. If intraoperative histological and immunohistochemical findings suggest a diagnosis of pancreatic hamartoma, a minimal pancreatic resection can be performed, sparing the patient the unnecessary risk of postoperative complications associated with major resections [26].

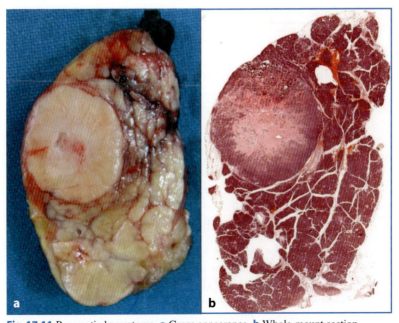

Fig. 17.11 Pancreatic hamartoma. **a** Gross appearance. **b** Whole-mount section

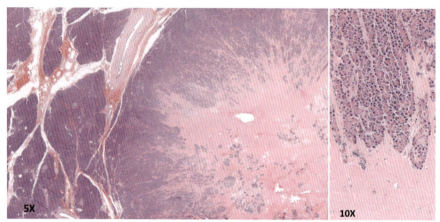

Fig. 17.12 Pancreatic hamartoma at histologic examination as seen at different magnifications: well-circumscribed lesion composed of disorganized acini with central fibroblastic, heavily collagenized stroma

17.4   Intrapancreatic Accessory Spleen

Intrapancreatic accessory spleen (IPAS) is a congenital anomaly that is due to the fusion failure of splenic primordial mesenchymal tissues, mimicking, in some case, a pancreatic neoplasm. A large study of approximately 3000 autopsies concluded that 10–12% of the populations examined had an accessory spleen. Most (80%) are situated in the adipose tissue at the splenic hilum, followed by the pancreatic tail (17%). Other, uncommon sites are the wall of the jejunum, mesentery, and pelvis [27].

Usually, IAPS are resected because they are misdiagnosed by imaging as pancreatic neoplasms. At ultrasonography, they appear as well-defined, usually well vascularized lesions [28]. On contrast-enhanced CT or MRI, the contrast enhancement of IAPSs at the arterial and portal phases is more intense than that of normal pancreatic parenchyma, simulating a pancreatic neuroendocrine neoplasm (PanNEN) [29-31]. The usefulness of octreotide scintigraphy is very limited for the differential diagnosis of IPAS and PanNEN, because splenic tissue, and in particular the white pulp, typically also expresses somatostatin receptors [32].

Three cases of resected IPAS have been seen at our institution. Interestingly, two of the three patients had undergone splenectomy for abdominal trauma some years before the finding of the IPAS, suggesting that a compensatory hyperplasia of the accessory splenic tissue may result in these tumor-like lesions. Therefore, in the case of a hypervascularized well-circumscribed nodule within the pancreatic tail (Fig. 17.13) in a patient who has previously undergone splenectomy, it is very important to distinguish IPAS from PanNENs, to avoid unnecessary surgery.

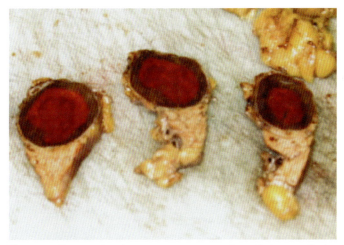

Fig- 17.13 Heterotopic spleen: gross appearance of a well-circumscribed nodule of red splenic tissue surrounded by normal pancreas

Accordingly, in our opinion IPAS should be suspected in the presence of hypervascular lesions located in the tail of the pancreas, in patients who have previously undergone splenectomy.

References

1. Yoshida K, Toki F, Takeuchi T et al (1995) Chronic pancreatitis caused by an autoimmune abnormality. Proposal of the concept of autoimmune pancreatitis. Dig Dis Sci 40:1561-1568
2. Chari ST, Kloeppel G, Zhang L et al (2010) Histopathologic and clinical subtypes of autoimmune pancreatitis: the Honolulu consensus document. Pancreas 39:549-554
3. Zamboni G, Luttges J, Capelli P et al (2004) Histopathological features of diagnostic and clinical relevance in autoimmune pancreatitis: a study on 53 resection specimens and 9 biopsy specimens. Virchows Arch 445:552-563
4. Sah RP, Chari ST, Pannala R et al (2010) Differences in clinical profile and relapse rate of type 1 versus type 2 autoimmune pancreatitis. Gastroenterology 139:140-8
5. Maire F, Le Baleur Y, Rebours V et al (2011) Outcome of Patients With Type 1 or 2 Autoimmune Pancreatitis. Am J Gastroenterol 106:151-156
6. Kamisawa T, Kim MH, Liao WC et al (2011) Clinical characteristics of 327 Asian patients with autoimmune pancreatitis based on Asian diagnostic criteria. Pancreas 40:200-205
7. Frulloni L, Scattolini C, Falconi M et al (2009) Autoimmune pancreatitis: differences between the focal and diffuse forms in 87 patients. Am J Gastroenterol 104:2288-2294
8. Kim HM, Chung MJ, Chung JB (2010) Remission and relapse of autoimmune pancreatitis: focusing on corticosteroid treatment. Pancreas 39:555-560
9. Finkelberg DL, Sahani D, Deshpande V et al (2006) Autoimmune pancreatitis. N Engl J Med 355:2670-2676
10. Manfredi R, Graziani R, Cicero C et al (2008) Autoimmune pancreatitis: CT patterns and their changes after steroid treatment. Radiology 247:435-443

11   Frulloni L, Amodio A, Katsotourchi AM et al (2007) A practical approach to the diagnosis of autoimmune pancreatitis. World J Gastroenterol 17:2076-2079

12   Shimosegawa T, Chari ST, Frulloni L et al (2011) International consensus diagnostic criteria for autoimmune pancreatitis: guidelines of the International Association of Pancreatology. Pancreas 40:352-358

13.   Neoptolemos J, Bhutani M (2006) Fast Facts: Diseases of the Pancreas band Biliary tract, Health Press, Oxford, UK, pp 77-92

14.   Stolte M, Weiss W, Volkholz H, Rösch W (1982) A special form of segmental pancreatitis: "groove pancreatitis. Hepatogastroenterology 29:198-208

15.   Becker V, Mischke U (1991) Groove pancreatitis. Int J Pancreatol 10:173-182

16.   Adsay NV, Zamboni G (2004) Paraduodenal pancreatitis: a clinico-pathologically distinct entity unifying "cystic dystrophy of heterotopic pancreas", "para-duodenal wall cyst", and "groove pancreatitis". Semin Diagn Pathol 21:247-254

17.   Fékété F, Noun R, Sauvanet A (1996) Pseudotumor developing in heterotopic pancreas. World J Surg 20:295-298

18.   Colardelle P, Chochon M, Larvol L et al (1994) Cystic dystrophy in an antro-duodenal heterotopic antroduodenal pancreas. Gastroenterol Clin Biol 18:277-280

19.   Procacci C, Graziani R, Zamboni G et al (1997) Cystic dystrophy of the duodenal wall: radiologic fi ndings. Radiology 205:741-747

20.   Zamboni G, Capelli P, Scarpa A et al (2009) Nonneoplastic Mimickers of Pancreatic Neoplasms. Arch Pathol Lab Med 133:439-453

21.   Itoi T, Sofuni A, Itokawa F et al (2011) Current status of diagnostic endoscopic ultrasonography in the evaluation of pancreatic mass lesions. Dig Endosc 1:17-21

22.   Yoshinaga S, Suzuki H, Oda I, Saito Y (2011) Role of endoscopic ultrasound-guided fine needle aspiration (EUS-FNA) for diagnosis of solid pancreatic masses. Dig Endosc 1:29-33

23.   Casetti L, Bassi C, Salvia R et al (2009) "Paraduodenal" pancreatitis: results of surgery on 58 consecutives patients from a single institution. World J Surg 33:2664-2669

24.   Nagata S, Yamaguchi K, Inoue T et al (2007) Solid pancreatic hamartoma. Pathol Int 57:276-280

25.   Pauser U, Kosmahl M, Kruslin B et al (2005) Pancreatic solid and cystic hamartoma in adults: characterization of a new tumorous lesion. Am J Surg Pathol 29:797-800

26.   Pauser U, da Silva MT, Placke J et al (2005) Cellular hamartoma resembling gastrointestinal stromal tumor: a solid tumor of the pancreas expressing c-kit (CD117). Mod Pathol 18:1211-1216

27.   Halpert B, Gyorkey F (1959) Lesions observed in accessory spleens of 311 patients. Am J Clin Pathol 32:165-168

28.   Dodds WJ, Taylor AJ, Erickson SJ et al (1900) Radiologic imaging of splenic anomalies. AJR Am J Roentgenol 155:805-810

29.   Gayer G, Zissin R, Apter S et al (2001) CT findings in congenital anomalies of the spleen. Br J Radiol 74:767-772

30.   Harris GN, Kase DJ, Bradnock H, Mckinley MJ (1994) Accessory spleen causing a mass in the tail of the pancreas: MR imaging findings. AJR Am J Roentgenol 163:1120-1121

31.   Schreiner AM, Mansoor A, Faigel DO, Morgan TK (2008) Intrapancreatic accessory spleen: mimic of pancreatic endocrine tumor diagnosed by endoscopic ultrasound-guided fine-needle aspiration biopsy. Diagn Cytopathol 36:262-265

32.   Suriano S, Ceriani L, Gertsch P et al (2011) Accessory spleen mimicking a pancreatic neuroendocrine tumor. Tumori 97:39e-41e

Index

A
Acinar cell
  carcinoma (ACC) 159
  cystadenoma (ACA) 28
Adenosquamous carcinoma 149
Anaplastic carcinoma 155
Autoimmune pancreatitis (AIP) 193, 194

C
Colloid carcinoma 153
Contrast-enhanced ultrasound (CEUS) 80-83
Cystadenocarcinoma 29
Cystic endocrine neoplasms 29

E
European neuroendocrine tumor society
  (ENETS) 74

G
Gastrinoma 65, 100
Gastro-entero-pancreatic neuroendocrine
  tumors (GEP)NENs 135
Germ-cell tumors 170
Glucagonoma 67, 101
Granular cell tumor (GCT) 168

H
Hepatoid carcinoma 167

I
Imaging findings 81, 86, 93

I
Insulinoma 64, 99
Intraductal papillary mucinous neoplasms
  (IPMN) 33
  epidemiology 34
  genetics 39
  pathology 34

symptoms 40
treatment 44
  branch-duct 46
  combined 47
  main duct 44
  postoperative follow-up 48
Intrapancreatic accessory spleen 204
Intraoperative ultrasound (IOUS) 81

L
Lymphoepithelial cysts 29

M
Malignant cystic neoplasms 53
  oncologist diagnosis and management 54-56
Mature teratoma 29
Medullary carcinoma 155
Mesenchymal tumors
  benign 189
  malign 190
Mucinous cystic neoplasms (MCN) 15
  diagnostic imaging 16, 17
  differential diagnosis 19
  pathology 18
  symptoms 16
  treatment 21
Multidetector computed tomography (MDCT)
  84, 87-89
Multiple endocrine neoplasia type 1 (MEN1)
  71, 75, 113

N
Neuroendocrine pancreatic neoplasms
  (PanNENs) 59
  chemotherapy 137
  classification 71
  epidemioloy 61
  functioning 71
    diagnostic strategies 102

imaging features 98
genetics 75
inherited 62
imaging 79
  computed tomography 84
  magnetic resonance imaging 91
  ultrasound 80
non-functioning 63
  diagnostic strategies 103
nuclear medicine imaging 121
  octreoscan imaging 121, 123, 124, 126
pathology 72
peptide receptor radionuclide therapy
(PRRT) 126
radiopharmaceuticals 118-120
staging and grading 74
surgical therapy 109
  laparascopic approach 113
  localized PanNENS 110
  locally advanced PanNENs 111
  metastatic PanNENs 112
targeted therapies 138
  PI3k-Akt-mTOR pathway 138
Neurofibromatomosis type 1 (NF1) 71, 75
Non-epithelial tumors 189

P

Pancreatic
  hamartoma 203
  metastasis 175
    clinicopathological features 175
Pancreatoblastoma 162
Paraduodenal pancreatitis 199
Primary non-epithelial tumors 189
Primary pancreatic lymphoma 165

R

Renal cell carcinoma 179
  diagnosis 180
  pathology 184
  symptoms 179
  treatment 181
    medical 183
    surgical 181

S

Serous cystic adenoma (SCA) 5
  diagnostic imaging 6-8
  pathology 9
  symptoms 5
  treatment 12
Serous cystoadenocarcinoma 12
Solid papillary neoplasms (SPNs) 4
  diagnostic imaging 26
  pathology 24
  symptoms 25
  treatment 27
Somatostatin
  analogues 103, 118-123, 125, 129
  receptors (SSTRs) 117-124
Somatostatinoma 67, 101
Sugar tumors 171

T

Tuberous sclerosis complex (TSC) 71, 75
Tumor-like lesions 183

V

VIPoma 66, 101
Von Hippel-Lindau (VHL) syndrome 6, 71, 75

Z

Zollinger-Ellison syndrome (ZES) 65

Printed in September 2012